Medication Administration Workbook

Lena L. Deter, MPH, RN

Educational Translator
DELHEC, LLC
Educational Services and Consulting

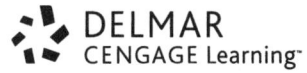

Australia • Brazil • Japan • Korea • Mexico • Singapore • Spain • United Kingdom • United States

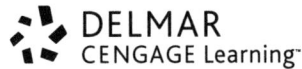

Medication Administration Workbook, First Edition
Lena L. Deter, MPH, RN

Vice President, Career and Professional Editorial: Dave Garza

Director of Learning Solutions: Matthew Kane

Acquisitions Editor: Matt Seeley

Managing Editor: Marah Bellegarde

Product Manager: Laura J. Wood

Editorial Assistant: Samantha Zullo

Vice President, Career and Professional Marketing: Jennifer Baker

Marketing Director: Wendy E. Mapstone

Senior Marketing Manager: Kristin McNary

Marketing Coordinator: Scott A. Chrysler

Production Director: Carolyn Miller

Senior Art Director: Jack Pendleton

© 2011 Delmar, Cengage Learning

ALL RIGHTS RESERVED. No part of this work covered by the copyright herein may be reproduced, transmitted, stored, or used in any form or by any means graphic, electronic, or mechanical, including but not limited to photocopying, recording, scanning, digitizing, taping, Web distribution, information networks, or information storage and retrieval systems, except as permitted under Section 107 or 108 of the 1976 United States Copyright Act, without the prior written permission of the publisher.

> For product information and technology assistance, contact us at
> **Cengage Learning Customer & Sales Support, 1-800-354-9706**
> For permission to use material from this text or product,
> submit all requests online at **www.cengage.com/permissions**.
> Further permissions questions can be e-mailed to
> **permissionrequest@cengage.com**

Library of Congress Control Number: 2010930030

ISBN-13: 978-1-4354-8173-2

ISBN-10: 1-4354-8173-9

Delmar
5 Maxwell Drive
Clifton Park, NY 12065-2919
USA

Cengage Learning is a leading provider of customized learning solutions with office locations around the globe, including Singapore, the United Kingdom, Australia, Mexico, Brazil, and Japan. Locate your local office at: **international.cengage.com/region**

Cengage Learning products are represented in Canada by Nelson Education, Ltd.

To learn more about Delmar, visit **www.cengage.com/delmar**
Purchase any of our products at your local college store or at our preferred online store **www.cengagebrain.com**

Notice to the Reader
Publisher does not warrant or guarantee any of the products described herein or perform any independent analysis in connection with any of the product information contained herein. Publisher does not assume, and expressly disclaims, any obligation to obtain and include information other than that provided to it by the manufacturer. The reader is expressly warned to consider and adopt all safety precautions that might be indicated by the activities described herein and to avoid all potential hazards. By following the instructions contained herein, the reader willingly assumes all risks in connection with such instructions. The publisher makes no representations or warranties of any kind, including but not limited to, the warranties of fitness for particular purpose or merchantability, nor are any such representations implied with respect to the material set forth herein, and the publisher takes no responsibility with respect to such material. The publisher shall not be liable for any special, consequential, or exemplary damages resulting, in whole or part, from the readers' use of, or reliance upon, this material.

Printed in the United States of America
1 2 3 4 5 6 7 14 13 12 11 10

Table of Contents

To the Learner / v

SECTION 1   REVIEW ACTIVITIES AND CLINICAL APPLICATIONS

Module 1   Ethical and Legal Aspects

Chapter 1   Introduction to Medication Administration   5
Chapter 2   Regulatory Issues   10
Chapter 3   Ethical and Legal Issues   14

Module 2   Medication Fundamentals

Chapter 4   Introduction to Medications   23
Chapter 5   Medication Orders   30
Chapter 6   Principles of Medication Administration   45

Module 3   Medication Administration

Chapter 7   Administration of Nonparenteral Medications   59
Chapter 8   Administration of Oxygen   70
Chapter 9   Administration of Enemas   85
Chapter 10   Care and Use of Gastrostomy and Jejunostomy Tubes   93
Chapter 11   Administration of Epinephrine by EpiPen   102

Module 4   Medications and Their Effects on the Body

Chapter 12   Body Organizations and Systems   111
Chapter 13   Vitamins, Minerals, and Herbs   129
Chapter 14   Topical Medications   134
Chapter 15   Eye and Ear Medications   140
Chapter 16   Psychotropic Medications   143
Chapter 17   Analgesics and Anesthetics   148

Chapter 18 Antiparkinsonian Medications, Anticonvulsants, and Medications for Treating Alzheimer's Disease   154
Chapter 19 Medications for Treating Infections   158
Chapter 20 Medications for Treating Cancer   165
Chapter 21 Medications for Treating Cardiovascular Disorders   170
Chapter 22 Medications for Treating Endocrine Disorders   175
Chapter 23 Medications for Treating Gastrointestinal Disorders   180
Chapter 24 Medications for Treating Musculoskeletal Disorders   185
Chapter 25 Medications for Treating Respiratory Disorders   189
Chapter 26 Medications for Treating Urinary Disorders   193
Chapter 27 Medications for Treating Reproductive System Disorders   197

Module 5 Communication and Documentation

Chapter 28 Role of the Unlicensed Assistive Personnel (UAP) in Medication Administration   203
Chapter 29 Transcription of Licensed Health Care Provider Orders   211

Module 6 Safety

Chapter 30 Additional Considerations   239
Chapter 31 Poison Control   248

Module 7 Additional Knowledge and Skills

Chapter 32 Basic Math   257
Chapter 33 Vital Signs   263
Chapter 34 Care of Individuals with Epilepsy   272
Chapter 35 Substance Abuse   280

SECTION 2 PERFORMANCE RECORD AND SKILL CHECKLISTS

To The Learner

This workbook was created especially for you. Its purpose is simple: to offer you the opportunity to practice the knowledge and skills that you have recently learned. If you allow it to, the workbook will take you through different clinical settings and scenarios. The workbook provides you with hands-on experience with the various tasks involved in safe and effective medication administration. The workbook also serves to reinforce the knowledge that you have recently gained.

To help you learn, the workbook uses a variety of questions and clinical applications. The questions and clinical applications follow the outline of its respective chapter. The book also includes skill checklists. The skill checklists provide you with a step-by-step guide to the procedures you must learn.

The information needed to answer all of the questions in this workbook may be found in the textbook, *Medication Administration,* ISBN-10: 1-4354-8172-0, by Lena Deter.

It is the author's hope that this workbook will offer each learner the encouragement and support needed to become successful with medication administration.

SECTION 1
Review Activities and Clinical Applications

MODULE 1
Ethical and Legal Aspects

Chapter 1
Introduction to Medication Administration

Learning Objectives

After completing the exercises in this chapter, you should be able to:
1. Spell and define terms.
2. Briefly describe the development of institutional care in the United States.
3. Describe three changes in health care in the United States over the past 40 years.
4. List three goals of deinstitutionalization.
5. List five settings in which a UAP might work.
6. Explain three purposes of the Nurse Practice Act.
7. Describe four models of nursing care.
8. List the five rights of delegation.
9. Explain the two choices a UAP has when a task is assigned to him.

INTRODUCTION

The exercises you complete in this chapter will address the following key concepts from the textbook chapter:

- the development of institutional care in the United States
- changes in health care in the United States over the past 40 years
- deinstitutionalization
- settings in which a UAP might work
- oversight and supervision
- various models of nursing care
- the Nurse Practice Act
- delegation

VOCABULARY

Define the following terms.

1. Adult Foster Care _____
2. assisted living facility _____
3. hospice _____
4. "least restrictive setting" _____
5. long-term care facility _____
6. supportive housing _____

COMPLETION

Complete the following statements by filling in the blanks.

7. In the late 18th and early 19th centuries, care was given to ill or disabled individuals in places called _____.

8. When hospitals were first built, the individuals cared for had _____ and _____.

9. When hospitals were first built, individuals with _____ and _____ were not allowed in for treatment.

10. In the 20th century, _____ were built to care for individuals with infectious diseases.

11. In the 20th century, state governments built _____ to care for individuals with mental illness and _____.

12. Deinstitutionalization is the process of _____.

13. According to the American Association on Mental Retardation, the three factors that define mental retardation are:

    a. _____
    b. _____
    c. _____

14. List the three goals of deinstitutionalization.
    a. _____
    b. _____
    c. _____

MATCHING

Draw lines to connect the terms in the left column with their definitions in the right column.

15. Medicare
16. Medicaid
17. Nurse Practice Act
18. scope of practice
19. multidisciplinary team
20. delegation

a. the legal act of assigning tasks or duties
b. the legal limits within which an individual may work
c. money from the federal government that the states use to pay for the care of individuals who have no money of their own
d. a government program that partially pays for health care for individuals over the age of 65 or who are permanently disabled
e. regulates nursing practice within each state
f. a team of professionals and paraprofessionals who work together to provide care to an individual and his family

CHOICES

21. From the choices below, circle five settings in which a UAP might work.

    full-time residential program   hospital
    fire station   work day treatment program
    EMT station   hospice
    rest home   correctional facility
    crisis intervention program

22. From the choices below, circle three purposes of the Nurse Practice Act.
    a. To protect the health, welfare, and safety of the citizens living in the state
    b. To allow the nurse to pass most of her job duties on to a UAP
    c. To determine the tasks a UAP may perform
    d. To define the scope of practice for licensed nurses
    e. To allow the nurse to practice her skills on coworkers

PICK THE CORRECT TERM

From the following list, pick the correct term to complete each definition in questions 23 to 28.

    functional nursing   primary care nursing

    team nursing   case management

    total patient care   professional oversight

23. When a staff of only registered nurses (RNs) is assigned to provide all of the care needed by a group of patients, this is called _____.

24. When an RN organizes the services of a multidisciplinary team and may or may not provide direct care, this is called _____.

25. When assignments are made by a charge nurse according to the type of task and the work to be done, this is called _____.

26. When one RN has the total responsibility of managing nursing care for a specific group of patients for the entire 24-hour period of hospitalization, including writing and supervising the plan of care, and associate RNs or licensed practical nurses (LPNs) on other shifts carry out the plan of care, this is called _____.

27. When the RN or LPN organizes the activities or duties of the licensed staff and UAPs to provide care for a group of patients, this is called _____.

28. When an RN provides monitoring of the medication administration program and practices of medication-certified UAPs, this is called _____.

COMPLETION

Complete the following statements by filling in the blanks.

29. List the Five Rights of Delegation. Provide brief descriptions of each "right."

    a. _____

    b. _____

    c. _____

    d. _____

    e. _____

30. When a nurse assigns a task to the UAP, what are the UAP's choices? _____

31. List the UAP's responsibilities when she accepts a task.

CHOICES

32. From the choices below, circle five reasons why a UAP may refuse a task.
   a. The UAP does not like to do the task assigned to him.
   b. The task is beyond the UAP's scope of function.
   c. The UAP is not trained to do the task safely.
   d. The UAP does not agree with the nurse's decision.
   e. The UAP does not know how to use the equipment or supplies.
   f. The nurse's directions are unclear or incomplete.
   g. The UAP does not want to do the task assigned to him.
   h. The nurse's request is illegal, unethical, or against policy.

SUMMARY

Because of the controls put into place by the United States government over the past years, our health care system has changed the way care is provided. In the past, individuals were cared for in hospitals for long periods of time. Today individuals experience short hospital stays. Healing occurs more often at home. Death may occur at home. The need for UAPs has grown greatly over the years. Their tasks and duties have changed and continue to change. Medication administration by UAPs is one of these changes.

Chapter 2
Regulatory Issues

Learning Objectives

After completing the exercises in this chapter, you should be able to:

1. Spell and define terms.
2. Explain the three purposes of the Pure Food and Drug Act of 1906.
3. Name two oversight agencies that deal with medications and drugs.
4. List five of the rules from the Federal Food, Drug and Cosmetic Act of 1938 with their amendments of 1951 and 1965.
5. List four of the rules of the Controlled Substances Act, which was written to set tighter controls on a specific group of drugs and medications.
6. Give two examples of each of the five schedules of drugs/medications.
7. Explain how state laws may differ from federal laws.
8. List the three legal terms used for medications and explain how they differ from each other.

INTRODUCTION

The exercises you complete in this chapter will address the following key concepts from the textbook chapter:

- federal laws pertaining to medication administration and controlled substances
- state laws pertaining to medication administration and controlled substances

VOCABULARY

Define the following terms.

1. drug standards _____
2. pharmaceutical company _____
3. schedules _____
4. controlled substances _____

COMPLETION

Complete the following statements by filling in the blanks.

5. Drug standards ensure that all medications called by the same name must have the same _____, _____, and _____.

6. According to the drug standards, a pharmaceutical company must not add other _____ or other _____ to a medication.

7. In 1906, the federal government passed a law to protect our supply of food and medications. This was called the _____.

8. There were two other issues addressed by this same law. List the two other issues.
   a. _____
   _____
   b. _____
   _____

9. Two oversight agencies were created by the federal government in the mid-1900s. They were the _____ and the _____.

10. In 1938 the federal government passed a law to prevent tampering with medication, food, and cosmetics. This was called the _____.

11. List the seven rules established in that act.

a. _____
b. _____
c. _____
d. _____
e. _____
f. _____
g. _____

12. In 1970 the federal government passed a law that set tighter controls on a specific group of medications that were being abused by society. This law is called the _____ _____

13. List the six rules established by that act.

a. _____
b. _____
c. _____
d. _____
e. _____
f. _____

14. Controlled substances are grouped into _____ schedules.

15. Controlled substance schedules are based on _____ and _____.

16. Schedule C-I drugs, such as heroin, have the potential to be the _____ dangerous and are _____ likely to be abused.

17. Schedule C-V drugs, such as Robitussin AC cough syrup, pose the _____ danger and are _____ likely to be abused.

18. Describe three symbols that indicate that a medication is a controlled substance.

a. _____
b. _____
c. _____

19. Each state can follow federal laws regarding medication, or the state may _____.

20. The UAP is responsible for knowing _____ and _____ guidelines for medication administration, handling, and storage.

21. List six differences among states that the UAP might see regarding medications.

a. _____

b. _____

c. _____

d. _____

e. _____

f. _____

SUMMARY

Federal laws regulate medication handling, storage, and administration across the country. State laws regulate medication handling, storage, and administration within each state. It is the UAP's responsibility to know his own state regulations, as well as federal guidelines for the safe and effective handling, storage, and administration of medications.

Chapter 3
Ethical and Legal Issues

Learning Objectives

After completing the following exercises, you should be able to:

1. Spell and define terms.
2. List the three health care documents regarding an individual's rights and describe six items these documents have in common.
3. Describe the difference between ethical standards and legal standards.
4. List three ethical principles that are important to the UAP.
5. Describe the role of an ethics committee.
6. List the basic rules for sharing information.
7. Describe various legal theories.
8. Describe the four elements of negligence.
9. Explain three legal situations that UAPs should avoid.

Chapter 3 Ethical and Legal Issues

INTRODUCTION

The exercises you complete in this chapter address the following key concepts from the textbook chapter:

- common health care documents regarding an individual's rights
- ethical standards and legal standards to be followed by the UAP
- the role of an ethics committee in the UAP's workplace
- guidelines for appropriate sharing of an individual's medical information
- various legal theories that are related to the UAP's role as a caregiver
- elements of negligence in the UAP's role as a caregiver

VOCABULARY

Define the following terms.

1. informed consent _____
2. advance directive _____
3. grievance _____
4. ethical standards _____
5. legal standards _____
6. liable _____
7. criminal liability _____
   _____
8. civil liability _____
   _____
9. discrimination _____
   _____
10. negligence _____
    _____
11. duty _____
12. breach _____
13. causation _____
    _____
14. statute of limitations _____
    _____
15. *Respondeat Superior* _____
    _____
16. comparative negligence _____
    _____
17. malpractice _____
    _____

MATCHING

Draw lines to connect the terms in the left column with its definition in the right column.

18. Omnibus Budget Reconciliation Act
19. Resident's Bill of Rights
20. Patient Care Partnership: Understanding Expectations, Rights, and Responsibilities
21. Client's Bill of Rights

a. describes the basic rights to which an individual is entitled while in a hospital or outpatient clinic

b. states the rights of an individual receiving home health care

c. states the rights of residents living in long-term care facilities

d. regulates the education and certification of nursing assistants in long-term care facilities

COMPLETION

Complete the following statements by filling in the blanks.

22. There are three types of Bill of Rights documents used in health care settings. While each one is written for a different group of individuals receiving health care, all documents emphasize the rights of the client, resident, or patient. List six rights all clients, residents, and patients have.

   a. _____
   b. _____
   c. _____
   d. _____
   e. _____
   f. _____

23. In her job, the UAP will need to make decisions about her actions. The two sets of rules that will guide the UAP as she makes her decisions are _____ and _____.

24. Ethical standards are guides to _____ behavior.

25. Legal standards are guides to _____ behavior.

26. When ethical standards are not followed, the UAP fails to live up to the promise to give _____, _____ care, and to do _____ _____.

27. Failing to live up to ethical standards may result in _____.

28. When legal standards are not followed, the UAP may be _____ and found _____ for injury or damage.

29. Failing to follow legal standards may result in _____ of _____, and/or _____, and/or _____.

30. Not following ethical or legal standards could also result in _____ of _____ and inability to _____ in the health care field.

QUESTIONS

Using what you have learned from the textbook, answer these questions.

31. In general, how may the UAP protect herself from liability when doing her job?

_____
_____

32. In the health care field, there are individuals from many different professions, as well as family members who all care for and about an individual. At times, these individuals may not agree on the best way to care for this individual. What is one way in which these disagreements may get settled?

_____
_____

33. What is the job of the ethics committee? How does this committee do its job?

_____
_____
_____
_____

34. Robert is a man with Lou Gehrig's disease. He has been living at a long-term care facility for the last 12 years. All of the staff members know him well. He has talked to you more than anyone else about how his quality of life has gone down in the last couple of years. He is tired of the constant poking, prodding, and interventions that need to be done to keep him alive. Robert recently told his doctor that he wants his feeding tube removed. The doctor wants Robert to keep his feeding tube in place. What information could you share that would be helpful to the ethics committee in this situation?

_____
_____
_____
_____
_____

35. Describe the Health Insurance Portability and Accountability Act of 1996, also known as HIPAA.

_____
_____
_____

36. How does HIPAA affect the UAP in her daily work? _____

_____
_____

COMPLETION

Complete the following.

37. List six guidelines the UAP should follow according to HIPAA when she is sharing information about the individual(s) in her care.

   a. _____
   b. _____
   c. _____
   d. _____
   e. _____
   f. _____

38. List six rules the UAP should follow to avoid legal problems at work.

   a. _____
   b. _____
   c. _____
   d. _____
   e. _____
   f. _____

39. Give two examples of statutes that apply to a UAP's daily work.

   a. _____
   b. _____

40. List the four elements of negligence.

   a. _____
   b. _____
   c. _____
   d. _____

CLINICAL APPLICATIONS

Read the following clinical scenarios. Using what you have learned from the textbook, answer the questions that follow each scenario.

41. When you are on your lunch break, a coworker approaches you. She says that her mother knows Mrs. Goldberg, an individual in your care. She asks how Mrs. Goldberg is doing, saying that her mother wanted to know. What should you do?

   _____

42. Mr. Pearson's minister comes to you after visiting Mr. Pearson. He says that some of the congregation members are asking about Mr. Pearson's recent treatments and test results. He says, "I wonder if you could give me a brief update on his health and prognosis." What should you say? _____

   _____

43. Deborah is working as a UAP in a group home. One of her assigned tasks for her shift is to check that the front door is locked after 9 p.m. because a resident named Phil has a history of leaving the home and wandering at night. Deborah gets a personal call at 8:45 p.m. and forgets to check the front door. Phil leaves the home at 9:10 p.m. Phil trips in the front yard and sprains his ankle. What type of legal issue is this?

44. Gary works as a UAP in a rest home. He is alone in a resident's room when he sees some videotapes on the shelf. He figures that no one will notice if just one is missing, so he chooses one and takes it home. What type of legal issue is this?

45. Sarah works at the same rest home as Gary does. Sarah sees Gary taking the videotape from the resident's room. Gary tells Sarah that if anyone asks her what happened, she would say that Gary borrowed it. What should Sarah do?

46. If she does nothing, what type of legal issue is that?

47. Lila is a UAP at a day program. One of the clients, Robert, is sitting at a table when he suddenly begins to shout. This causes Lila to spill a pitcher of water and some pills. She yells, "Robert, you idiot, look what you made me do! If you don't shut up, I'll call the cops on you, I mean it!" What type of legal issue is this?

48. Sam is a UAP at a group home. He is giving care to Albert. Without warning, Albert punches him in the stomach. Sam grabs Albert's arm and pushes him to the floor. Albert hits his head and gets a cut on his forehead.
    a. What type of legal issue is this?
    b. What could Sam have done that would have been a safer response?

49. Violet is physically handicapped and requires help to feed herself. Steve, a UAP, is trying to feed her lunch. Violet keeps complaining about everything, from the food to the way Steve is feeding her. Steve finally says, "Okay, Violet, if that's how you're going to be, then what if you just skip lunch today? In fact, I won't give you dinner either. How does that sound?" He takes her away from the table and parks her wheelchair in the corner where Violet is separated from the rest of the individuals in the room. She cannot move her chair and begins to cry.
    a. What type or types of legal issues are these?
    b. Is there more than one type of legal issue in this situation?
    c. What could Steve do that would be a better response?

50. What must the UAP do if she suspects that an individual in her care is being abused?

51. Mr. Jovio lives at a long-term care facility. He has identified himself as a homosexual. During a.m. care, Sarah makes a negative comment to Mr. Jovio about his sexual orientation. Sarah also refuses to give Mr. Jovio any additional care. Mr. Jovio reports Sarah's comment to the administrator of the facility. Is this negligence or discrimination? Why? _____

_____

_____

52. Lucy is a UAP who has made it quite clear to her colleagues that she does not like individuals of Hispanic origin. Mr. Hernandez comes from Puerto Rico. Lucy has to give care to Mr. Hernandez. She helps Mr. Hernandez to the toilet, gives him the string for his call light, and says that she will be back in a few minutes. While Lucy is assisting another resident, Mr. Hernandez gets up from the toilet by himself. He falls in the bathroom and breaks his arm. Is this negligence or discrimination? Why?_____

_____

_____

53. John is a UAP who is working in a facility that is new to him. While giving medications, he gives Mrs. Yakowitz a medication that was ordered for Mrs. Sakowitz. Is this negligence or discrimination? Why? _____

_____

_____

54. Sam is a UAP who is known for getting his work done as quickly as possible, even if it is not the best work he can do. His supervisor has been doing documentation audits in the last month. She has noticed on three separate audits that Sam documents the care he gives before he has done it. There have been no complaints from the individuals Sam gives care to. Can Sam's supervisor discipline Sam for this? Why or why not? _____

_____

_____

55. a. In example 51, could Sarah be sued for malpractice? Why or why not?

_____

  b. In example 52, could Lucy be sued for malpractice? Why or why not?

_____

_____

_____

SUMMARY

As a caregiver, the UAP has a responsibility to follow ethical and legal standards when giving care. If the UAP has any questions or finds herself in a difficult situation, the UAP should talk with her supervisor to be sure that she is following appropriate standards of care. If the UAP observes a coworker doing something that is unethical or illegal or that violates the rights of an individual in her care, the UAP should report it to her workplace supervisor. Following ethical and legal standards will help to ensure that the UAP does her job safely and gives the best care possible.

MODULE 2
Medication Fundamentals

Chapter 4
Introduction to Medications

Learning Objectives

After completing the exercises in this chapter, you should be able to:
1. Spell and define terms.
2. Identify four types of medication names.
3. Explain the difference between the brand or trade name and the generic name. Give examples of each.
4. Describe the three basic types of medication preparation.
5. List five types of semisolid and solid medications.
6. List five types of liquid medications.
7. Describe three of the main therapeutic actions of medications.
8. Explain the difference between a side effect, an adverse reaction, and a medication interaction.
9. List the factors a licensed health care provider takes into consideration when prescribing a medication.
10. Choose the medication reference book or material that would be easiest to use.

INTRODUCTION

The exercises you complete in this chapter will address the following key concepts from the textbook chapter:

- types of medication names
- three basic types of medication preparation
- main therapeutic actions of medications
- side effects, adverse reactions, and medication interactions
- factors a licensed health care provider takes into consideration when prescribing a medication
- medication reference materials

VOCABULARY

Define the following terms.

1. pharmacology _____
2. drug _____
3. generic equivalents _____
4. drug substitution laws _____
5. dosage _____
6. dose _____
7. idiosyncrasies _____
8. pediatric clients _____
9. geriatric clients _____

MATCHING

A drug is a substance used in medicine that may affect how the body works. There are six uses for these drugs, also called medications. Six of the uses for drugs are listed on the left. Draw a line to connect each type of drug/medication use in the left column with its description in the right column. The descriptions may be used more than once.

10. therapeutic use
11. diagnostic use
12. curative use
13. replacement use
14. preventative use
15. prophylactic use

a. medication used to prevent or lessen the severity of a disease
b. medication used to replace substances normally found in the body
c. medication used in the treatment of disease
d. medication that kills or removes the cause of a disease
e. medication used in radiology

Most medications have four names. The types of medication names are listed on the left. Draw a line to connect each type of medication name in the left column with its description in the right column.

16. generic name
17. trade name
18. chemical name
19. official name

a. the molecular formula for the medication
b. the name of the medication as it appears in the USP/NF
c. the formal name by which the medication is marketed and sold
d. the common or general name of the medication

COMPLETION

Complete the following sentences by filling in the blanks.

20. The generic name of a medication is written with a _____, never capitalized.

21. The trade name of a medication is _____ and is only used by one pharmaceutical company.

22. The trade name of a medication is written with a _____, not a lowercase letter like the generic name.

23. The trade name of a medication is also called the _____ of a medication.

24. The symbol _____ is usually found after the brand name of the medication on a label. This symbol means that the name is a _____.

25. The official name of a medication is usually the same as _____ of the medication.

26. Generic and brand names of medications can be compared to the various names of grocery products. Give two examples of generic grocery names that are not listed in the textbook.

   a. _____
   b. _____

   Give two examples of a brand name for each of those generic names.

   1. _____
   2. _____
   1. _____
   2. _____

27. When a pharmaceutical company develops a new medication, it must be tested and approved by the FDA. After the FDA approves the medication, the company has the exclusive right to sell the medication for _____ years.

28. Why would a generic equivalent medication be helpful to an individual?
_____

29. Give two reasons why a licensed health care provider would choose not to give his patient a generic equivalent drug.
   a. _____
   b. _____

30. If a licensed health care provider chooses to give his patient a brand name medication rather than a generic equivalent, he must write _____ on the prescription.

CHOICES

31. From the list below, circle the types of liquid medications.

emulsion	tablet	caplet	solution
capsule	suspension	mixture	troche
syrup	lozenge	elixir	tincture
ointment	lotion	aerosol	suppository
liniment	spray	topical	

32. From the list below, circle the types of solid and semisolid medications.

tablet	spray	elixir	mixture
ointment	emulsion	troche	liniment
suppository	aerosol	solution	suspension
capsule	topical	lozenge	caplet
tincture	syrup	lotion	

MATCHING

One type of solid medication is a tablet. On the left is a list of different types of tablets. Match each type of tablet on the left with its description on the right.

33. enteric-coated   a. dissolves in the vagina
34. buccal   b. is chewed and then swallowed
35. sublingual   c. has two or more layers of medication
36. chewable   d. dissolves in the small intestine
37. effervescent   e. dissolves under the tongue
38. vaginal   f. has a groove or slit cut into its surface
39. layered   g. releases active ingredients when placed in water
40. scored   h. dissolves in the mouth between the cheek and gum

MATCHING

Draw lines to connect each phrase in the left column with its definition on the right.

41. selective action
42. agonist action
43. antagonist action
44. local action
45. remote action
46. specific action
47. systemic action

a. external medication acts on the part of the body where it is applied
b. medication has a particular effect on certain bacteria or other pathogens
c. medication mixes with special sites on specific cells to cause a response
d. medication is absorbed into the bloodstream and is carried throughout the body, affecting all the cells
e. medication blocks the effect of a second medication
f. medication acts on certain body tissues or a specific body part
g. medication acts on a part of the body away from where it is given

COMPLETION

Complete the following statements by filling in the blanks.

48. A side effect is _____ that may _____ of the medication.

49. Give an example of a medication side effect that is not listed in the textbook.
    _____

50. An adverse reaction is _____ that is _____.

51. Give an example of a medication adverse reaction that is not in the textbook.
    _____

52. A medication interaction is _____. It may occur with substances other than a medication, including _____, _____, _____, and _____.

53. Give an example of a medication interaction. _____
    _____

54. When prescribing or ordering a medication, the licensed health care provider may consider many different factors. List eight factors he must consider.

    a. _____
    b. _____
    c. _____
    d. _____
    e. _____
    f. _____
    g. _____
    h. _____

28 Module 2 Medication Fundamentals

55. Pediatric clients do not take the same dosage of medication as adults. This is because _____.

56. The geriatric client group is not divided into different age groups because _____.

57. In addition to the factors listed in number 54, the licensed health care provider may consider special factors when prescribing medication for a geriatric client. List those special factors.

   a. _____
   b. _____
   c. _____
   d. _____
   e. _____
   f. _____
   g. _____
   h. _____

MATCHING

A dose of medication is the amount that is ordered for administration. In other words, it is the amount that an individual gets each time he is given the medication. On the left is a list of terms for different doses. Draw a line to connect each term in the left column with its description in the right column.

58. initial dose
59. average dose
60. maintenance dose
61. maximum dose
62. minimum dose
63. therapeutic dose
64. divided dose
65. unit dose
66. lethal dose
67. toxic dose

a. the amount of medication that causes signs and symptoms of poisoning
b. the amount of medication that could kill an individual
c. portions of the dose given over a period of time
d. a premeasured amount of medication, individually packaged
e. the amount of medication that is most effective and has the least amount of side effects
f. the first dose given of a medication
g. the amount of medication needed to keep a therapeutic level in an individual's bloodstream
h. the smallest amount of medication that will be effective
i. the largest amount of medication that may safely be given
j. the amount of medication needed to produce the desired effect

REFERENCE LISTS

68. List three reference books that may be used by the UAP to gather information on medications.

a. _____

b. _____

c. _____

69. List four Internet Web sites that are reliable professional sources of medication information.

a. _____

b. _____

c. _____

d. _____

70. Why is it important to use only those Web sites that are under the authority of the government and/or supervised by professional groups when the UAP is gathering medication information? _____

_____

_____

SUMMARY

The UAP should have a basic knowledge of medications. Being able to identify the medications' names, the classification of medications with their therapeutic actions, the uncommon actions of medications, and the factors used to determine the amount of medications an individual receives allows the UAP to administer medications safely and effectively. Reference materials provide an ongoing means of support for the UAP.

Chapter 5
Medication Orders

Learning Objectives

After completing the exercises in this chapter, you should be able to:
1. Spell and define terms.
2. List the eight parts of a medication order.
3. Briefly describe the five most common types of medication orders.
4. Explain the difference between a written order and a verbal order.
5. List the seven guidelines to follow when taking a telephone order.
6. Describe three of the most common forms used in medication administration.
7. Describe two types of health care provider order forms.
8. Describe Computerized Physician Online Entry (CPOE).
9. Describe an Electronic Medication Administration Record (eMAR).
10. Explain the difference between the manufacturer's label for a prescription medication, the prescription label from the pharmacy, and the label on an over-the-counter medication.
11. Explain the importance of following a time schedule for medication administration.

INTRODUCTION

The exercises you complete in this chapter will address the following key concepts from the textbook chapter:

- the parts of a medication order
- the different types of medication orders
- the forms used in medication administration
- reading and completion of the following forms:
  - medication sheet
  - HCP order forms
  - telephone order forms
- Computerized Physician Online Entry (CPOE)
- use of an Electronic Medication Administration Record (eMAR)
- reading a manufacturer's label
- reading a pharmacy label
- reading an OTC medication label
- setting time schedules for giving medications

VOCABULARY

Define the following terms.

1. medication orders _____
2. routine order _____
3. single order _____
4. standing order _____
5. stat order _____
6. prn order _____
7. written orders _____
8. verbal orders _____
9. telephone orders _____
10. faxed orders _____
11. prescription _____
12. over-the-counter (OTC) medication _____

COMPLETION

Complete the following statements by filling in the blanks.

13. A medication order is a written _____ from the _____ to the _____ .

14. Medication orders are written by the licensed health care provider for a specific individual. Each medication order contains eight parts. List the eight parts.

   a. _____
   b. _____
   c. _____
   d. _____
   e. _____
   f. _____
   g. _____
   h. _____

15. Each medication order should follow a specific sequence. The _____ is written first. The _____, _____, and _____ are written next.

MATCHING

Read each medication order. Under each order, draw lines to connect the word or phrase in the left column with the correct word or phrase in the right column.

Order: Motrin 400 mg by mouth q4h

16. Motrin   a. frequency to be given
17. 400 mg   b. route to be given
18. by mouth   c. name of the medication
19. q4h   d. dose of the medication

Order: Lanoxin 0.25 mg by mouth daily

20. Lanoxin   a. route to be given
21. 0.25 mg   b. frequency to be given
22. by mouth   c. dose of the medication
23. daily   d. name of the medication

Order: Vicks Formula 44 10 mL by mouth q6h

24. Vicks Formula 44   a. dose of the medication
25. 10 mL   b. name of the medication
26. by mouth   c. frequency of the medication
27. q6h   d. route to be given

MATCHING

Read each licensed health care provider order. Draw lines to connect the licensed HCP order in the left column with the type of order in the right column.

28. Diflucan 150 mg
    1 tab by mouth once in AM

29. Zoloft 50 mg
    1 tab by mouth bid

30. Tylenol 325 mg
    2 tabs by mouth q4h for headache

31. nitroglycerin 0.3 mg
    1 tab sublingual by mouth stat

32. Robitussin 10 mL
    by mouth q4h prn for cough

a. standing order
b. stat order
c. prn order
d. single order
e. routine order

QUESTIONS

Read each question. Using what you have learned from the textbook, answer each question with one or two phrases or sentences.

33. How does the licensed health care provider give a written order?

    _____

34. Why is a written licensed HCP order the best type of medication order?

    _____

35. If the UAP has a question about a written medication order or if the written order is not readable, what must the UAP do? _____

    _____

    _____

36. How does the licensed health care provider give a verbal order?_____

    _____

37. If a licensed health care provider wants to give a verbal medication order to the UAP, what should the UAP do?_____

    _____

    _____

38. How does the licensed health care provider give a telephone order?

    _____

34 Module 2 Medication Fundamentals

39. If the UAP is allowed to take a telephone order, what are the seven guidelines she should follow when taking the telephone order?

   a. _____
   b. _____
   c. _____
   d. _____
   e. _____
   f. _____
   g. _____

40. If the UAP takes a telephone order from the licensed HCP, how does the order get signed?

   _____
   _____

41. How does the licensed health care provider give a faxed order?

   _____

42. How is a prescription different from a medication order?

   _____
   _____

43. It is the responsibility of the UAP to understand the information on the medications that the licensed health care provider is ordering. List two methods the UAP might find helpful to increase her understanding of the medications.

   a. _____
   b. _____

44. Should the UAP give a medication if she does not understand a medication order?

   _____

45. If not, who may the UAP ask for assistance?

   _____

46. What should the UAP do if she is confused or unsure about the medication order?

   _____
   _____

47. Who may the UAP ask if she has questions about a specific medication, such as whether it may be taken with food?

   _____

48. When the UAP is checking the medication sheet before giving a medication, what should she specifically check for?

   _____

Chapter 5 Medication Orders

MEDICATION ADMINISTRATION FORMS

This section includes samples of common forms the UAP may see at her work site.

Figure 5-1 is a sample of a health care provider (HCP) order form that may be used in an institutional setting such as a hospital or a nursing home. Using what you have learned from the textbook, read the HCP form (Figure 5-1). Answer the questions below.

49. What is the individual's name? _____

50. What are the date and time the orders were written?
_____

51. Does the individual have any allergies? If so, what is she allergic to?
_____

52. What medications did the licensed health care provider order?
_____

53. What is the licensed health care provider's name?
_____

Figure 5-2 is a sample of an HCP order form that may be used in a community setting. The top section has been filled in by the individual's UAP. The bottom section has been completed by the licensed health care provider. Using what you have learned from the textbook, read the HCP form (Figure 5-2). Answer the questions below.

54. What is the individual's name? _____

55. What is the date of the visit to the licensed HCP? _____

56. Does the individual have any allergies? If so, what is he allergic to?
_____

57. What is the name of the licensed health care provider? _____
_____

58. Why did the UAP take this individual to see his licensed HCP? _____
_____
_____

59. What medications is he currently taking? _____
_____
_____

60. What are the findings of the licensed HCP? What is meant by this? _____
_____
_____

61. What are the medication or treatment orders to treat this problem?
_____
_____
_____

| Medical Center Hospital
Physician's Order Sheet
Instructions:
1. Imprint the patient's identification plate onto the form before placing form into the chart.
2. After each set of orders are written, remove the first yellow copy and send it to the pharmacy.
3. "X" out the remaining unused lines after the last yellow copy is used. | Mary Highlander
DOB 4/16/1953
126 Main Street
Westchester, IL 63506 |

ALLERGIES sulfa drugs

Date Ordered	Time Ordered	Time Executed	Time Posted	Use Ball Point Pen Only
5/1/10	10:00 AM			alprazolam (Xanax) 2 mg 1 tab by mouth bid. Notify licensed HCP if pt c/o insomnia or tension headaches.
				cimetidine (Tagamet) 400 mg 1 tab by mouth at bedtime. *Dr. Steven Jones* ~~~~~~~

Figure 5-1 Health Care Provider's Order Form used in an institutional setting *(Delmar/Cengage Learning)*

Health Care Provider Order Form	
Name : Paul O'Rourke	Date : 6/15/11
Health Care Provider : Dr. Mary Stone	Allergies : NKA
Current Medical/Dental Conditions : Epilepsy	
Reason for Visit : Paul has been complaining of right ear pain for the last 2 days. He also spiked a fever last night of 102.6°F.	
Current Medications : Zoloft 50 mg by mouth tid, Ativan 2 mg by mouth bid, Dilantin 100 mg by mouth tid	
Staff Signature : Sarah Kowalski, UAP	6/15/11
Findings by Health Care Provider : Upon examination, Mr. O'Rourke is in mild distress and is holding his right ear. Otoscopic exam done bilaterally, with significant redness and fluid build-up in the right middle ear. Mr. O'Rourke exhibits symptoms of otitis media in his right ear.	
Medications/Orders : cephalexin (Keflex) 500 mg one tab by mouth q6h x 10 days	
Instructions : Finish entire prescription. Notify Dr. Stone if pt. continues to c/o right ear pain after 3 days or if pt. develops a rash.	
Follow-Up Visit : 6/28/11	Lab Work/Tests : none
Health Care Provider Signature : Dr. Mary Stone	Date : 6/15/11

Figure 5-2 Health Care Provider's Order Form commonly used in a community setting *(Delmar/Cengage Learning)*

62. Are there any special instructions or precautions for the medications or treatments?

   _____

   _____

63. Is a follow-up visit or lab work needed? If so, give the specifics of the follow-up visit and/or lab work.

   _____

Here is a sample of a medication sheet. This medication sheet lists specific information about a medication that has been ordered by the licensed health care provider. Using what you have learned from the textbook, read the form and answer the questions that follow.

Medication or Treatment		Hours	1	2	3	4	5	6	7	8	9	10	11	12	13	14	15
Start	Generic Digoxin																
	Brand Lanoxin																
Stop	Strength 0.25 mg																
	Amount 1 tab																
	Frequency daily in AM																
	Route By mouth																
Special Instructions/Precautions:																	

(Delmar/Cengage Learning)

64. There are two names given for the medication. What are they?

_____

65. What is the strength of the medication? _____

66. What is the frequency of the medication to be given?

_____

67. What is the route of the medication to be given?

_____

Figure 5-3 is a sample of a telephone order form. This form may be used as a guideline for the UAP when gathering information during a phone conversation with a licensed health care provider. The form is to be signed by the licensed HCP after it is completed. Once signed, the order then becomes a legal order. Using what you have learned from the textbook, read the sample telephone order form (Figure 5-3). Answer the questions that follow.

Telephone Order Form	
Date of Telephone Order : May 2, 2009	**Time of Order :** 10:30 AM
Name of the Individual : Samantha Connors	

Name of Medication :	
Generic : dexchlorpheniramine	**Brand :** Dexchlor

Strength : 2 mg
Amount : 1 tablet
Frequency : q6h
Route : by mouth
Reason for Medication Being Ordered or for Change in Medication Order : Pt. has been taking Bromfenex, an OTC antihistamine/decongestant, for seasonal allergies with rhinitis. However, she has recently developed more severe symptoms including urticaria.
Special Instruction or Precautions : Notify licensed HCP if hives continue after 3 days or if pt. does not get relief of allergy symptoms in 3 days.
Instructions for Refused or Forgotten Medication : If one dose is missed, may give one dose within 2 hours of the missed dose. If more than one dose is missed, call licensed HCP for instructions.
Discontinue Date (if any) : D/c Bromfenex 2 tabs po tid on 5/2/09
Health Care Provider's Name : Dr. James Proctor

Staff Signature/Title : Ronald Tuttle, UAP	**Co-Signature of Staff/Title :** Paul Leonard, UAP
Signature of Health Care Provider : James Proctor, MD	**Date :** 5/3/09

Figure 5-3 Sample Telephone Order Form *(Delmar/Cengage Learning)*

68. What are the date and time that the telephone order was taken by the UAP?

_____

_____

69. What is the name of the individual who will be getting the medication or treatment?

_____

_____

70. What is the reason for the new or changed medication? _____
_____

71. Is there a medication that will be discontinued? If so, what is it?
_____

72. Write the name, strength, dose, frequency, and route of the new medication. _____
_____
_____

73. Are there any special instructions for giving this medication? If so, what are they?
_____
_____

74. Did the licensed HCP give instructions for any common side effects that may occur? If so, what are the side effects and instructions? _____
_____
_____

75. What should the UAP do if the medication is refused or forgotten?
_____
_____

76. Is there a discontinue date? If so, what is the date?
_____

77. What is the name of the licensed health care provider giving this order?
_____

78. What is the name of the UAP who took this order?
_____

What is the name of the UAP who cosigned the order? _____

ELECTRONIC MEDICAL RECORD

79. An electronic medical record includes many sections including the _____ and an _____.

80. _____ is a computerized, organized method by which licensed health care providers are able to enter (write) orders for the treatment of individuals.

81. To prevent medication errors and ensure safety, the Joint Commission and the Institute for Safe Medication Practices (ISMP) recommend that workplaces use the _____ to document and track medication administration.

82. The _____ is a computerized record that eliminates all paper records and creates an organized system for medication administration.

LABELS

This section includes samples of a manufacturer's label, a prescription label, and an over-the-counter (OTC) medication label.

Below is a sample of a manufacturer's label for a prescription medication. Study the label carefully. Fill in the blanks that follow.

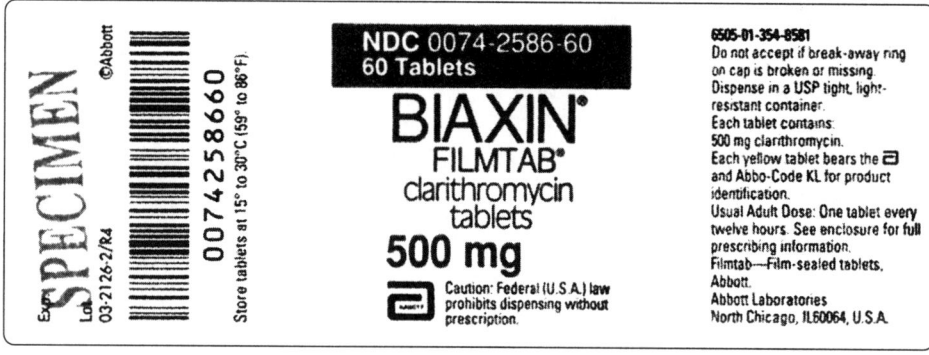

(Delmar/Cengage Learning)

83. The trade or brand name for the medication is _____.

84. The generic name is _____.

85. The National Drug Code (NDC) number is _____.

86. The strength in a given amount of the medication is _____.

87. The usual dose and frequency of administration are _____.

88. The form in which the medication is supplied is _____.

89. Warnings or cautionary statements include _____.

90. The expiration date of the medication is _____.

91. The lot or batch code is _____.

92. The manufacturer's name and address are _____.

93. The total number and/or volume of medication in the container is _____.

Below is a sample of a prescription label. Study the label carefully, then fill in the blanks that follow.

Rx: 135246   Acme Pharmacy   (231)555-0987
                        25 Main Street
                        Livingston, NY 54321

Carlson, David   Date filled: 4/16/10

V-Cillin K 250 mg   Qty: 40 tablets
penicillin V potassium

Directions for use: Take one tablet by mouth every 6 hours for 10 days. Finish all medication unless directed otherwise by physician.

Dr. James Proctor
lot #9944500   exp. date: 6/2011   refills: 0

(Delmar/Cengage Learning)

94. The prescription number is _____.

95. The name, address, and telephone number of the pharmacy are _____ _____.

96. The name of the individual for whom the medication is ordered is _____.

97. The date the prescription is filled is _____.

98. The brand name of the medication is _____.

99. The generic name of the medication is _____.

100. The strength of the medication is _____.

101. The amount of medication in the bottle is _____.

102. Directions for use are _____ _____.

103. The lot number is _____.

104. The expiration date of the medication is _____.

105. The name of the licensed health care provider is _____.

106. The number of refills is _____.

Below is a sample of an OTC medication label. Study the label carefully. Fill in the blanks that follow.

Dad's Pink Pills Antacid

Active ingredients:
bismuth subsalicylate 525 mg
antidiarrheal, upset stomach reliever

50 chewable tablets

- calms upset stomach
- soothes heartburn
- relieves diarrhea

Directions for use
Chew 1–2 tablets every
4–6 hours as needed
to relieve symptoms.

Inactive ingredients:
red #4, flavor, aluminum silicate,
saccharin sodium, methylparaben,
sorbic acid, citric acid.

Warnings: Contains salicylate. Do not take if you are allergic to salicylates (such as aspirin) or if you are taking other salicylate products.

exp. date 4/2011
lot# 35746809

Acme Medical, Inc.
Cleveland, TN 24685

(Delmar/Cengage Learning)

107. The brand name of the medication is _____.

108. The generic name of the medication is _____.

109. The total amount of the medication in the container is _____.

110. List the active ingredients and their purposes. _____.

111. The inactive ingredients are _____.

112. List three of the uses of this medication. _____.

113. The directions for taking this medication are _____.

114. Warnings and cautionary statements are _____.

115. The name and address of the manufacturer are _____

_____.

116. The expiration date of this medication is _____.

117. The lot number is _____.

COMPLETION

Complete the following statements by filling in the blanks.

118. When giving medications, it is important to follow a time schedule. Times of administration for routine medications are important for two reasons. List the two reasons.

   a. _____

   b. _____

119. Whenever possible, it is important to schedule medication administration so that an individual's _____ is disturbed as little as possible.

120. Fill in the empty boxes in the chart below.

Abbreviation	What it means	Sample schedule
daily		
	twice a day	
		8 AM, 2 PM, 8 PM
qid		
	at bedtime	
		12 AM, 4 AM, 8 AM, 12 PM, 4 PM, 8 PM
q6h		

(Delmar/Cengage Learning)

SUMMARY

Medication orders are written instructions from the licensed health care provider to the UAP. The UAP must be able to read and interpret information on medication orders, medication labels, and various forms used in the workplace. Understanding this information is essential for giving safe and effective care.

Chapter 6
Principles of Medication Administration

Learning Objectives

After completing the exercises in this chapter, you should be able to:

1. Spell and define terms.
2. Define the "Six Rights" of medication administration.
3. Describe the Three Checks.
4. Explain the formula "dose = strength × amount."
5. List five of the basic guidelines for medication administration.
6. List seven occasions when the UAP should wash his hands.
7. Describe three situations when gloves are worn for medication administration.
8. Describe the four steps in the procedure for medication administration.
9. Provide a description of a medication room and storage area.
10. Complete documentation for a Controlled Substance Count.
11. State three reasons for disposing of a medication.
12. State acceptable methods for disposing of a medication.
13. Complete documentation for disposing of a medication.

INTRODUCTION

The exercises you complete in this chapter will address the following key concepts from the textbook chapter:

- the basic steps and guidelines for medication administration
- administration of medications safely and effectively
- handwashing
- documentation of controlled substances
- disposal of medications
- the UAP's legal responsibility to administer medications as he has been trained and according to the policies and regulations within the setting where he works

VOCABULARY

Define the following terms.

1. dose _____
2. strength _____
3. amount _____
4. internal medication _____
5. external medication _____

COMPLETION

Complete the following statements by filling in the blanks.

6. When the UAP is making sure that he is giving medication to the right individual, he can identify the individual by _____ or by _____.

7. Once the UAP has identified the right individual, he must then compare the individual's name on the following three documents to make sure the name matches before he can give the medication: a) _____, b) _____, and c) _____.

8. To make sure that he is giving the right medication, the UAP checks the name of the medication in three places to make sure the name of the medication matches in all three places before he gives the medication. These three places are as follows:

    a) _____, b) _____, and
    c) _____.

9. The right dose of medication is written in the _____. The right dose is equal to _____ × _____.

10. Before the UAP gives a medication, he must compare the dose to be given with the dose ordered on the _____, and the dose on the _____ _____, and lastly the dose on the _____.

11. The right time to give a medication may mean:

    a. _____

    b. _____

    c. _____

    d. _____

12. The UAP may give a medication _____ before it is due, to _____ after it is due, in order to follow the licensed health care provider's order.

13. The right time must be checked in three places before the UAP can give a medication. These are: a) _____, b) _____, and c) _____.

14. The route of a medication is _____.

15. Before giving a medication, the UAP must check the route on three documents to make sure all three match. These documents are: a) _____, b) _____, and c) _____.

16. Each time the UAP checks one of the Six Rights, he must _____ to avoid errors before giving the medication.

17. Describe the Three Checks including the documents used for each check.

    a. _____

    b. _____

    c. _____

18. The Three Checks are made to go together with the _____.

MATCHING

Draw lines to connect each abbreviation in the left column with the definition in the right column.

19. daily   a. every four hours
20. bid   b. three times a day
21. tid   c. every eight hours
22. q4h   d. every day
23. q6h   e. every six hours
24. q8h   f. twice a day

Draw lines to connect each word in the left column with its matching word in the right column.

25. *I*   a. dose
26. *Must*   b. route
27. *Do*   c. individual
28. *This*   d. medication
29. *Right*   e. time

PROBLEM SOLVING

Using the formula, "dose = strength × amount," solve the following problems.

30. The licensed health care provider's order says *Coumadin 5 mg by mouth daily.* Coumadin 2.5-mg tablets are available. Give _____ tablets.

31. The licensed health care provider's order says *Motrin 600 mg by mouth bid.* Motrin 300-mg tablets are available. Give _____ tablets.

32. The licensed health care provider's order says *Lanoxin 0.125 mg by mouth daily.* Lanoxin 0.25-mg tablets are available. Give _____ tablets.

33. The licensed health care provider's order says *Lopressor 50 mg by mouth bid.* Lopressor 50-mg tablets are available. Give _____ tablets.

34. The licensed health care provider's order says *Urecholine 15 mg by mouth tid.* Urecholine 10-mg tablets are available. Give _____ tablets.

COMPLETION

Complete the following statements by filling in the blanks.

35. List five guidelines for giving medication. Explain why each guideline is important.

    a. _____

    b. _____

    c. _____

    d. _____

    e. _____

36. The single most effective way to prevent the spread of infection is to _____.

37. List seven occasions when the UAP should wash his hands.

    a. _____
    b. _____
    c. _____
    d. _____
    e. _____
    f. _____
    g. _____

38. List three situations in which the UAP needs to wear gloves.

a. _____

b. _____

c. _____

CHOICES

39. From the list below, choose three instances when gloves need to be changed.

a. after working with each individual on the UAP's assignment

b. after eating

c. after touching any item or surface that is soiled

d. before touching clean items or surfaces

e. between tasks with the same individual if there is contact with infectious material

f. after using the bathroom

CLINICAL APPLICATIONS

40a. Below is a list of the four specific steps that must be followed for medication administration to be done safely and correctly. Put them in the order in which they would be done by placing a number 1 next to the first step, a 2 next to the second step, and so on.

_____ Administration

_____

_____

_____ Documentation

_____

_____

_____ Preparation

_____

_____

_____ Begin by Pouring the Medication

_____

_____

40b. Under each step in number 40a above, describe what you would do for each step when administering medication.

41. Describe how a medication room should be set up.

42. Explain the four guidelines for medication storage.
   a.
   b.
   c.
   d.

QUESTIONS

Read the following questions. Using what you have learned from the textbook, answer each question with one or two phrases or short sentences.

43. What is another name for controlled substance medications?

44. There are two ways that staff members keep track of controlled substance medications. What are those ways?
   1.
   2.

45. Why must controlled substance medications be counted?

46. What is the name of the book in which the Controlled Substance Count is recorded?

47. List the three sections of a Controlled Substance Count Book. Describe each section.
   a.
   b.
   c.

CLINICAL APPLICATIONS

Figure 6-1 is a sample of a Controlled Substance Count Book index page. Study the page carefully and then answer questions 48 to 51.

INDEX

INDIVIDUAL'S NAME	MEDICATION & STRENGTH	PAGE NUMBER				SIGNATURE OF STAFF PERSON RESPONSIBLE FOR REMOVING MEDICATION FROM COUNT
Mary Sheehan	clonazepam 0.5 mg	1	7			
Mary Sheehan	diazepam 5 mg	2				
George Kowalski	butabarbital sodium 15 mg	3				
Sarah Killan	hydromorphone 2 mg	4				
Sarah Killan	chloral hydrate 500 mg	5				
Steven O'Reilly	alprazolam 1 mg	6	8			

**REMEMBER TO UPDATE INDEX INFORMATION WHEN ITEM IS TRANSFERRED TO ANOTHER PAGE.

Figure 6-1 Sample Index Page from a Controlled Substance Count Book *(Delmar/Cengage Learning)*

48. What controlled substance medications does Mary Sheehan take?

_____

49. On what pages are her medications documented? _____

_____

50. Who takes chloral hydrate? _____

51. On what pages are Steven O'Reilly's controlled substance medications documented?
_____

Figure 6-2 is a sample of a count page from the Controlled Substance Count Book. Study the page carefully. Answer questions 52 to 61.

Name: Gregory Kildare				( ) Original Entry or (x) Transferred from Page No. 22		
Licensed Health Care Provider: James Proctor		Pharmacy: Acme Pharmacy		Rx No. 3476298		Rx Date: 4/15/10
Drug & Strength: chlordiazepoxide (Librium) 10 mg				Rx No.		Rx Date:
Directions: Give two tablets 3 times a day.				Rx No.		Rx Date:

Date	Time	Amount on Hand	Amount Used	Route	Amount Left	Staff Signature
4/29/10	2:00 PM	20	2	po	18	Ronald Tuttle, UAP
4/29/10	8:00 PM	18	2	po	16	George Thomas, UAP
4/30/10	8:00 AM	16	2	po	14	Ronald Tuttle, UAP
4/30/10	2:00 PM	14	2	po	12	Ronald Tuttle, UAP
4/30/10	8:00 PM	12	2	po	10	George Thomas, UAP
5/1/10	8:00 PM	10	2	po	8	Paula Stefanopolis, UAP
5/1/10	10:30 AM	8	received 90		98	Paula Stefanopolis, UAP
5/1/10	2:00 PM	98	2	po	96	Paula Stefanopolis, UAP
5/1/10	8:00 PM	96	2	po	94	George Thomas, UAP
5/2/10	8:00 AM	94	2	po	94	Paula Stefanopolis, UAP
5/2/10	2:00 PM	94	2	po	92	Ronald Tuttle, UAP

MEDICATION DISCONTINUED/DISPOSED	MEDICATION TRANSFERRED
Discontinue Date: _____	New Page # _____
Removal Date: _____	
Signature Staff Removing: _____	Amount Transferred: _____
Signatures of Staff Destroying Medication: (2 signatures required) _____ _____	Signatures of Staff Verification: (2 signatures required) _____ _____

Figure 6-2 Sample Count Page from a Controlled Substance Count Book *(Delmar/Cengage Learning)*

52. Who is the individual who takes the medication documented on this page?

_____

_____

53. Who is the licensed health care provider? _____

54. What is the name of the pharmacy that provides this medication?

_____

55. What is the medication and its strength? _____

56. What are the directions for giving this medication?

_____

57. At what times was the medication given on 4/30/10?

_____

58. How many doses were available on 4/30/10, before the 2 p.m. dose was given?

_____

59. How many doses were available on 4/30/10, after the 8 p.m. dose was given?

_____

60. What happened on 5/1/10? _____

61. How many doses were available after that on 5/1/10? _____

_____

Figure 6-3 is a sample of a verification page from a Controlled Substance Count Book. Study the page carefully. Answer the questions 62 to 64.

62. Who did the Controlled Substance Count on 4/29/10 at 11 p.m.?

_____

63. Who verified that the count was correct on 4/29/10 at 11 p.m.?

_____

64. What times was the count done on 5/1/10? _____

To answer questions 65 and 66, refer to both the count page and the verification page of the Controlled Substance Count Book shown in Figure 6-3.

65. What happened on the date that the count was not correct? Explain the error.

_____

_____

_____

66. On your copy of the count page, correct the error that was made on 5/2/10. Also correct the count verification page.

_____

CONTROLLED SUBSTANCE COUNT VERIFICATION

DATE	TIME	COUNT CORRECT	STAFF COMING ON DUTY	STAFF GOING OFF DUTY
4/29/10	3:00 PM	yes	George Thomas, UAP	Ronald Tuttle, UAP
4/29/10	11:00 PM	yes	Samuel Livingston, UAP	George Thomas, UAP
4/30/10	7:00 AM	yes	Ronald Tuttle, UAP	Samuel Livingston, UAP
4/30/10	3:00 PM	yes	George Thomas, UAP	Ronald Tuttle, UAP
4/30/10	11:00 PM	yes	Samuel Livingston, UAP	George Thomas, UAP
5/1/10	7:00 AM	yes	Paula Stefanopolis, UAP	Samuel Livingston, UAP
5/1/10	3:00 PM	yes	George Thomas, UAP	Paula Stefanopolis, UAP
5/1/10	11:00 PM	yes	Samuel Livingston, UAP	George Thomas, UAP
5/2/10	7:00 AM	yes	Paula Stefanopolis, UAP	Samuel Livingston, UAP
5/2/10	3:00 PM	no	George Thomas, UAP	Paula Stefanopolis, UAP

Figure 6-3 Sample Verification Page from a Controlled Substance Count Book *(Delmar/Cengage Learning)*

QUESTIONS

Read each question. Using what you have learned from the textbook, answer each question with one or two phrases or short sentences.

67. All unused or discontinued medications must be destroyed. This process is called disposal of medications. List five reasons for medication disposal.

    a. _____
    b. _____
    c. _____
    d. _____
    e. _____

68. Steven O'Reilly goes out for a day trip with his family. When he leaves, a staff member gives his mother the medications that he is to take while he is gone. When he returns, his mother gives back the medication bottle with two pills inside and says, "Steve didn't want to take these. He said he can take them later on tonight." Is it okay to use these medications? _____
    _____

69. List five methods of destroying medications.

    a. _____
    b. _____
    c. _____
    d. _____
    e. _____

Figure 6-4 is a sample of a medication disposal documentation record. Study the form carefully. Answer questions 70 to 76.

Item # _____   Date last filled _7/23/10_

Name _Mary Sheehan_   Date _8/15/10_

Medication/strength _clonazepam 0.5 mg_

Rx # _0324589_   Pharmacy _Acme Medical_

Amount disposed _7_   Reason _Ms. Sheehan has transferred to another facility._

Controlled Substance Book # _3_   Page # _7_

Signatures: Staff member _Ronald Tuttle, UAP_

Supervisor _George Thomas, UAP_

Figure 6-4 Sample Disposal Form *(Delmar/Cengage Learning)*

70. What is the name of the individual who was taking the medication?
_____

71. What are the name and strength of the medication?
_____

72. When was the prescription for this medication last filled?
_____

73. How much of the medication was disposed of?
_____

74. What was the reason for the disposal? _____
_____

75. Where can the count for this medication be found?
_____

76. Who are the two staff members who disposed of the medication? _____
_____

SUMMARY

Safe and effective medication administration is based on a series of simple yet critical procedures and guidelines. These include:

- the Six Rights
- the Three Checks
- the basic guidelines for medication administration
- the four-step procedure for medication administration
- handwashing
- the use of gloves

Safe and effective medication administration also includes proper counting and documentation of controlled substances and disposal of unusable medications to guarantee that they are not being misused or abused.

MODULE 3
Medication Administration

Chapter 7
Administration of Nonparenteral Medications

Learning Objectives

After completing the exercises in this chapter, you should be able to:
1. Spell and define terms.
2. List three advantages and five disadvantages of taking medications orally.
3. Prepare medications for administration.
4. Demonstrate the administration of oral medications.
5. Demonstrate the administration of eye medications.
6. Demonstrate the administration of ear medications.
7. Demonstrate the administration of nasal medications.
8. Demonstrate the administration of transdermal medications.
9. Demonstrate the administration of rectal medications.
10. Demonstrate the administration of vaginal medications.
11. Demonstrate the application of medications to the skin and hair.
12. Demonstrate the use of an inhaler (MDI).
13. Demonstrate the use of a small-volume nebulizer and IPPB machine.
14. Write a clinical progress note for an individual receiving aerosol therapy.

Module 3 Medication Administration

INTRODUCTION

The exercises you complete in this chapter will address the following key concepts from the textbook chapter:

- nonparenteral routes of administration
- detailed procedures for administering medications
- equipment and supplies required for administration
- special considerations for administration of medications

VOCABULARY

Define the following terms.

1. parenteral medication _____
2. nonparenteral medication _____
3. oral medication _____
4. sublingual medication _____
5. topical medication _____
6. ophthalmic medication _____
7. otic medication _____
8. nasal medication _____
9. transdermal system _____
10. rectal medication _____
11. vaginal medication _____

COMPLETION

Complete the following statements by filling in the blanks.

12. The procedure for medication administration involves a series of steps. These steps are discussed in Chapter 6. List the four main steps of the procedure for medication administration.

    a. _____
    b. _____
    c. _____
    d. _____

13. When choosing the route of administration for an individual, the licensed health care provider may consider many different factors. List four of the factors the licensed HCP may consider.

    a. _____
    b. _____
    c. _____
    d. _____

14. Oral medications are the most common medications given. List three benefits of giving oral medications.

    a. _____
    b. _____
    c. _____

15. There are also disadvantages to giving oral medications. List four of these disadvantages.

    a. _____
    b. _____
    c. _____
    d. _____

16. Solid forms of oral medication include _____, _____, and _____.

17. Liquid forms of oral medication include _____, _____, and _____.

CHOICES

18. From the list below, circle the pieces of equipment that may be used in administering oral medications.

    | eMAR | medicine dropper | water-soluble lubricating gel |
    | medicine cup | paper tissue | drinking straws |
    | gloves | tablet crusher | face mask |
    | syringe | towel | medication tray |
    | cotton balls | water cup | medication sheet |

19. From the list below, circle the pieces of equipment that may be used in administering ophthalmic medications.

    | eMAR | sterile cotton balls | individual's eyedropper |
    | medicine cup | paper tissue | tablet crusher |
    | water cup | drinking straw | gloves |
    | medication sheet | syringe | |

20. From the list below, circle the pieces of equipment that may be used in administering rectal medications.

medication sheet	eMAR	water-soluble lubricating gel
towel	tablet crusher	water cup
syringe	medicine dropper	gloves
cotton balls	paper tissue	medicine cup

MATCHING

Draw lines to connect each term in the left column with its definition in the right column.

21. unit dose container
22. sterile
23. perforated eardrum
24. herpes
25. rebound congestion
26. scabies
27. pediculosis
28. suppository
29. inhaler
30. handheld inhaler

a. congestion caused by overuse of nasal sprays
b. sealed medication container that is under pressure
c. head lice
d. medication inserted into the rectum, vagina, or urethra
e. holds a single dose of medication
f. type of inhaler that is held in an individual's hand
g. free from bacteria
h. body lice
i. a hole in the ear drum
j. acute viral disorder

CLINICAL APPLICATIONS

Read the following paragraphs. Using what you have learned from the textbook, answer the questions.

You are asked to give Mr. Pakowski his morning medications. He takes four pills:

- digoxin 1 tab (0.125 mg)
- Ativan 1 tab (2 mg)
- aspirin 2 tabs (81 mg each tablet for a total of 162 mg)

He has also been recently diagnosed with an upper respiratory tract infection. For the upper respiratory tract infection he is taking:

- penicillin VK 2 tsp (250 mg total)
- Robitussin 2 tsp (200 mg total)

31. List the equipment you would use to give Mr. Pakowski his morning medications.

_____

_____

32. How would you prepare his medications?

_____

33. Which medications would you give first? _____

34. Which medication would you give last? Why? _____
_____

When you bring Mr. Pakowski his pills, he says that his throat is too sore to swallow them. He asks you to crush them. He says, "The girl last night gave me some applesauce to take my pills."

35. Where would the crushing of his medication be documented?
_____

36. Is it okay to crush Mr. Pakowski's pills? Why or why not?
_____

Once you recheck the licensed HCP orders, you see that the licensed HCP has given an order to crush Mr. Pakowski's pills and mix them with applesauce.

37. Name two different pieces of equipment you could use to crush the solid medications.
_____

38. How much applesauce should you use to give Mr. Pakowski his medications?
_____

39. Once you have given Mr. Pakowski his morning medications, what do you do next?
_____

Mrs. Johnson has an order for Naphcon-A. Naphcon-A is a type of eyedrop. It is an antibiotic and decongestant. You are asked to give her the midafternoon dose. The licensed HCP order calls for 2 drops to be given in each eye.

40. List the equipment you would use to give Mrs. Johnson her eyedrops.
_____
_____

41. What word or words should you see on the label of the eye medication container?
_____

42. After identifying Mrs. Johnson and preparing the medication, what is the first step in giving the eyedrops? _____
_____

43. Explain the correct use of an eyedropper. _____
_____

44. How should Mrs. Johnson be positioned in order for you to give her the eyedrops?
_____

45. What should you do if the drops go directly onto Mrs. Johnson's eye? _____
_____
_____

46. After you successfully administer the eyedrops, what should you do next?
_____
_____

64 Module 3 Medication Administration

47. What is the last step in giving an eye medication? _____
_____

Mr. Ledger has an order for Cipro HC Otic. Cipro HC Otic is a type of eardrops used to treat acute otitis externa, or "swimmer's ear." The licensed HCP order calls for three drops in the right ear, twice a day. The licensed HCP also orders a cotton ball to be placed in the ear after the drops are given. You are asked to give him his afternoon dose.

48. List the equipment you would use to give Mr. Ledger his eardrops.
_____
_____

49. When you approach Mr. Ledger to give him his eardrops, you notice that there is some drainage coming from his right ear. He is sticking his finger into the ear canal. What should you do? _____
_____
_____

50. How do you prepare Mr. Ledger's ear before you give the eardrops?_____
_____

51. How would you put the drops into the ear canal? _____
_____

52. After you give Mr. Ledger his eardrops, what else would you do to complete the procedure?_____
_____

53. What is the last step in giving an ear medication?
_____

Mrs. Hodgkins has an order for Astelin nasal spray. Astelin nasal spray is used to treat symptoms of seasonal allergies. The licensed HCP order calls for two sprays in each nostril twice a day. You are asked to give her morning dose.

54. List the equipment you would use to give Mrs. Hodgkins her nasal spray.
_____
_____

55. How would you position Mrs. Hodgkins to administer her nasal spray?
_____

56. How would you position Mrs. Hodgkins if you were giving nose drops instead of a spray? _____

57. What instruction would you tell her before giving the nasal spray?
_____

58. What is the last step in giving a nasal medication?
_____

Mr. Pelletier has an order for Absorbine Antifungal Foot Powder. Absorbine Antifungal Foot Powder is a type of powder used to treat a skin fungus sometimes called "athlete's foot." The licensed HCP order calls for a light layer of the powder to be applied twice a day. You are asked to give the evening dose.

59. List the equipment you would use to apply Mr. Pelletier's foot powder.

_____

_____

60. What piece of protective equipment must you use when administering the powder?

61. What steps will you need to complete before applying the powder to prepare Mr. Pelletier's skin? _____

_____

_____

62. How will you know how much powder to apply? _____

_____

63. What is the last step in applying a topical powder? _____

_____

After a few days of treatment, Mr. Pelletier's licensed HCP determines that the powder is not effective. He changes Mr. Pelletier's medication to Lamisil Cream. The licensed HCP order calls for the cream to be applied twice a day. You are asked to give the evening dose.

64. List the equipment you would use to apply Mr. Pelletier's foot cream.

_____

_____

65. How would you prepare his skin before applying the cream?

_____

_____

66. What is the difference in technique for applying a cream or ointment compared with applying a lotion or solution?

_____

_____

67. What is the last step in applying a topical cream?

_____

Mrs. Stone has an order for lindane shampoo. Lindane shampoo is used to treat pediculosis, or head lice. The licensed HCP order calls for 15 mL of shampoo to be applied and lathered for 4 to 5 minutes, then rinsed out of the hair. The licensed HCP order also states that the hair must be combed with a fine-tooth comb after shampooing to remove the nits.

68. List the equipment you would use to apply Mrs. Stone's shampoo.

_____

_____

66 Module 3 Medication Administration

69. Would you wash her hair first with a nonmedicated shampoo? Why or why not?
_____

70. Mrs. Stone has short hair. She usually lets it air dry after she washes it. Would you dry her hair with a hair dryer? Why or why not? _____
_____

71. The staff have been saying that other people living and working around Mrs. Stone may develop a case of head lice also. Mrs. Grady, another person living with Mrs. Stone, asks if she may borrow the medicated shampoo. What should you do? _____
_____
_____

72. What is the last step in applying a medicated shampoo?
_____

Mr. Billings has an order for a Nitro-Dur patch to be applied once a day for treatment of angina pectoris. You are asked to apply his patch.

73. List the equipment you would use to apply Mr. Billings's transdermal patch.
_____
_____

74. How would you let other staff members know when the patch was most recently changed? _____
_____

75. Why is it important to apply Mr. Billings's patch at the same time every day?
_____

76. A few hours after you apply Mr. Billings's patch while you are helping him change his shirt, you notice that his patch is gone. What do you do next?
_____
_____

77. What is the last step in applying a transdermal patch? _____
_____

Ms. Jennings has recently been complaining of constipation. She has not had a BM in three days. Her licensed HCP has ordered Bisacodyl Unisert, a rectal suppository. You are asked to give her the suppository.

78. List the equipment you would use to give Ms. Jennings a rectal suppository.
_____
_____

79. What instruction would you give Ms. Jennings before giving her the suppository?
_____

80. Describe how Ms. Jennings should be positioned for the administration of the suppository. _____

81. What instruction would you give Ms. Jennings after giving her the rectal suppository? _____

82. What is the last step in giving a rectal suppository? _____

Mrs. Berkowitz has vaginitis. Her licensed HCP has written an order for Sulfa-Gyn. Sulfa-Gyn is a vaginal cream that is an antibiotic. The licensed HCP order calls for applying one applicator full of cream twice a day. You are asked to give the evening dose.

83. List the equipment you would use to give Mrs. Berkowitz her vaginal medication. _____

84. What instruction would you give Mrs. Berkowitz before applying the vaginal cream? _____

85. How would you position Mrs. Berkowitz to apply the cream? _____

86. What do you need to look for before applying the cream? _____

87. Explain how to prepare and use the applicator for vaginal cream. _____

88. You must tell Mrs. Berkowitz two things after applying the vaginal cream. What are those two things? _____

89. What is the last step in applying a vaginal medication? _____

Mr. Thompson uses an inhaler, Azmacort Oral Inhaler, to control his asthma. The licensed HCP order for his inhaler calls for two inhalations three times a day. You are asked to give him his third dose of the day.

90. List the equipment you would use to give Mr. Thompson his inhaler. _____

91. What instructions would you give Mr. Thompson before giving him his inhalant medication? _____

92. Before giving the inhalant medication, you must remind Mr. Thompson to breathe out the stale air in his lungs. Why is it important that he only breathes out the stale air instead of emptying his lungs? _____

93. Why is it important for Mr. Thompson to brush his teeth and rinse with an oral rinse after using his inhaler? _____

94. List and describe the possible side effects from the overuse of inhalant medications. _____

95. What is the last step in giving an inhalant medication? _____

Mr. Brint receives a nebulizer treatment three times a day. This evening you will be helping Mr. Brint with his treatment.

96. What three steps must you perform before beginning Mr. Brint's treatment? _____

97. How long should you stay with Mr. Brint once his treatment begins? _____

98. List five possible side effects of a nebulizer treatment. _____

In your textbook there are three phrases used repeatedly in the directions for medication administration. Read each of the following phrases and write what it means.

99. "The principles and procedures for administering medications are always the same and are always followed." _____

100. "Complete steps 1 and 2 as per the procedure for giving medications." _____

101. "Complete step 4 as per the procedure for giving medications."
_____

SUMMARY

When administering medications, always remember the following:

- *Always* follow the Six Rights of medication administration, the Three Checks, and the procedure for giving each medication safely and effectively.

- Whenever there is a question about a medication or a procedure, *ask—ask* the supervisor, the pharmacist, or the individual's licensed health care provider—but *always* know the answer before giving a medication.

- *Never* use equipment until you have received the proper training and you are comfortable using the equipment.

- The UAP will most likely be the first person to see any changes in an individual who has received medication. *Always* report any changes to your supervisor and to the individual's licensed health care provider.

Chapter 8
Administration of Oxygen

Learning Objectives

After completing the following exercises, you should be able to:

1. Spell and define terms.
2. Explain the responsibilities of the UAP in regard to the administration of oxygen.
3. List five conditions that may require the administration of oxygen.
4. List eight signs and symptoms of an inadequate oxygen supply (hypoxemia).
5. Perform a pulse oximetry reading.
6. List six basic guidelines for the care of an individual who is receiving pulse oximetry.
7. List the four items that are to be included in the written licensed health care provider order for oxygen.
8. Describe the two most common methods of oxygen delivery.
9. Describe four types of oxygen administration equipment.
10. Demonstrate the changing of a prefilled humidifier bottle and a refillable humidifier bottle.
11. List ten basic guidelines for the care of an individual who is receiving oxygen.
12. Describe the four basic respiratory positions.
13. List five symptoms of oxygen toxicity.
14. Demonstrate the use of an incentive spirometer.
15. Demonstrate the use of a CPAP device.
16. Write a clinical progress note for an individual receiving:
    - pulse oximetry
    - incentive spirometer
    - CPAP
17. List six oxygen safety precautions.

INTRODUCTION

The exercises you complete in this chapter address the following key concepts from the textbook chapter:

- medical reasons for administering oxygen
- monitoring oxygen saturation levels using pulse oximetry
- procedures and equipment used for administering oxygen
- documenting the administration of oxygen
- use of an incentive spirometer
- use of a CPAP device
- recognizing signs and symptoms of oxygen toxicity

VOCABULARY

Define the following terms.

1. oxygen _____
2. congestive heart failure _____
3. COPD _____
4. cyanosis _____
5. dyspnea _____
6. hypoxemia _____
7. rales _____
8. atelectasis _____
9. hemoglobin _____
10. pulse oximeter _____
11. tracheostomy _____
12. oxygen concentrator _____
13. humidifier _____
14. incentive spirometer _____
15. CPAP device _____

QUESTIONS

Using what you have learned from the textbook, answer these questions.

16. Why would a licensed health care provider prescribe oxygen for an individual?
    _____
    _____

17. How can the UAP detect early signs of hypoxemia in a light-skinned individual?
    _____
    _____

18. How can the UAP detect early signs of hypoxemia in a dark-skinned individual?
    _____
    _____

19. What is pulse oximetry? _____
    _____
    _____

20. Which pulse oximeter sensors work best for a dark-skinned individual? _____
    _____
    _____

21. What major factor will interfere with the use of a pulse oximeter in all individuals?
    _____

22. Under what circumstance is the pulse oximeter *not* used? _____
    _____

23. The licensed health care provider has ordered a pulse oximeter for an individual. What question should the UAP always ask the licensed health care provider about the pulse oximeter alarm? _____

24. Why is it important to remove an individual's nail polish before placing a pulse oximeter sensor on the individual? _____
    _____
    _____

25. When removing an individual's nail polish, should the UAP remove the nail polish from only one finger or toe or from all of the individual's nails? _____
    _____

26. Under what circumstances may the UAP turn off the pulse oximeter alarm?
    _____

COMPLETION

Complete the following statements by filling in the blanks.

27. List five conditions that may require oxygen administration.

   a. _____
   b. _____
   c. _____
   d. _____
   e. _____

28. List eight signs and symptoms of hypoxemia.

   a. _____
   b. _____
   c. _____
   d. _____
   e. _____
   f. _____
   g. _____
   h. _____

29. Blood enters the _____ from the _____ through the _____ artery.

30. Once in the _____, the blood passes through tiny structures called _____.

31. In the alveoli, blood rids itself of _____ and picks up _____.

32. Oxygen is carried to the _____ of the body through the _____ by a part of the blood called _____.

33. List four types of pulse oximeter sensors.

   a. _____
   b. _____
   c. _____
   d. _____

34. A normal oxygen saturation level is between _____ and _____.

35. An oxygen saturation level below _____ may indicate complications.

36. Oxygen saturation levels below _____ need to be reported to the individual's licensed health care provider.

37. Readings below _____ are life threatening and require immediate attention.

38. For readings below 70%, the UAP must immediately call _____ or the _____.

MATCHING

Draw lines to connect each term in the left column with its definition in the right column.

39. congestive heart failure
40. COPD
41. kyphoscoliosis
42. Lou Gehrig's disease
43. multiple sclerosis
44. myocardial infarction
45. obesity
46. pneumonia
47. shock
48. sleep apnea

a. a state in which the body's circulation is disrupted and the blood pressure is dangerously low
b. a heart attack
c. a period of time during sleep when respirations stop for 10 seconds or more
d. an infection of the lungs
e. excess of fat in relation to lean body mass, with a body weight of 20% or more over ideal weight for height
f. a progressive disorder that destroys the motor nerves which control voluntary movement
g. failure of the heart to adequately pump blood throughout the body
h. a condition that interferes with normal breathing over a long period of time
i. a severe curvature of the spine
j. a disorder of the central nervous system caused by loss of myelin around central nervous system fibers

Draw lines to connect each term in the left column with its definition in the right column.

49. cyanosis
50. dyspnea
51. hypoxemia
52. rales
53. tachycardia

a. a moist respiration caused by fluid collecting in the air passages
b. a pulse of more than 100 beats per minute
c. a blue or purplish discoloration of the skin caused by a lack of oxygen
d. difficult or labored breathing
e. a condition in which there is a lack of oxygen in the blood

QUESTIONS

Using what you have learned from the textbook, answer these questions.

54. When using a pulse oximeter, what must the UAP do to prepare the sensor site?

_____

_____

_____

55. It is important for the UAP to make sure that the pulse oximeter is accurately measuring the individual's pulse rate. How does the UAP do this?

_____

_____

56. When setting up the pulse oximeter, it is important to cover the sensor with a towel or sheet? Why is this? _____

_____

57. When a pulse oximeter is being used for continuous monitoring, how often do clothespin-like sensors need to be moved to a new site? _____

_____

58. When using a pulse oximeter for continuous monitoring, how often do taped sensors need to be moved to a new site? _____

_____

59. Why is it important to change the position of the pulse oximeter sensor? _____

_____

_____

60. If the individual's pulse rate is different from the pulse rate being monitored by the pulse oximeter, what should the UAP do?

_____

_____

61. If the UAP notices a significant difference between current oxygen saturation levels and readings that were previously taken, what should the UAP do? _____

_____

_____

62. If an individual is receiving oxygen, what must the UAP do before applying the pulse oximeter? _____

_____

63. a. If a pulse oximeter sensor is taped in place on an individual's skin, what should the UAP do?

_____

_____

b. If the UAP notices signs or symptoms of an allergic reaction to the tape holding the sensor in place, what should the UAP do? _____

_____

_____

64. a. What is the problem with using a pulse oximeter on an individual who has thick fingernails or toenails? _____

_____

_____

b. What is one solution to this problem? _____

_____

_____

CLINICAL APPLICATIONS

A documentation sample for an individual receiving pulse oximetry follows. Read the progress note. Answer the questions that follow.

On 12/31/09 pulse oximetry is ordered for Mr. Smith by his licensed health care provider at 8:15 a.m.

Mr. Smith's progress note reads as follows:

12/31/09 8:30 AM Finger-clip sensor attached to left index finger. Sat level 92%, P 74 R 14 Color pale. Lips slightly cyanotic. Skin warm and dry to touch. Oxygen via n/c @ 2L/min.

12/31/09 9:00 AM Sat level 96% P 68 R 12 Lips, mucous membranes and nail beds pink.

65. At what time did Mr. Smith's licensed health care provider order a pulse oximetry reading? _____

66. At what time was the pulse oximeter sensor applied? _____

67. At what site was the sensor placed? _____

_____

68. a. What was the initial saturation rate? _____

b. What was the initial pulse rate? _____

c. What was the initial respiration rate? _____

69. What observations were made about Mr. Smith at the time the sensor was applied?

_____

_____

_____

70. a. Did Mr. Smith receive oxygen? _____

b. If Mr. Smith received oxygen, what was the flow rate? _____

c. If Mr. Smith received oxygen, how was it administered? _____

_____

71. At what time was the second pulse oximetry reading taken? _____

72. a. What was the saturation rate? _____

b. What was the pulse rate? _____

c. What was the respiration rate? _____

73. What observations were made about Mr. Smith at the time of the second pulse oximetry reading? _____

_____

_____

Samples of written licensed health care provider orders for oxygen therapy follow. Read each order. After each order, indicate what type of information is missing.

74. Order reads: *O_2 via nasal cannula when out of bed.*

Information missing: _____

_____

_____

75. Order reads: *O_2 3L/min 90% continuous.*

Information missing: _____

_____

_____

76. Order reads: *O_2 2L/min via mask.*

Information missing: _____

_____

_____

77. Order reads: *O_2 3L/min continuous.*

Information missing: _____

_____

_____

COMPLETION

Complete the following statements by filling in the blanks.

78. A nasal cannula is the _____ and _____ _____ method of oxygen delivery to use.

79. A nasal cannula is used to deliver _____ concentrations of oxygen to an individual.

80. A cannula is a long _____ that has two hollow, short tubes called _____.

81. The prongs are placed in the openings of the _____.

82. A mask is a _____ object that fits over an individual's _____, _____, and _____.

83. There is a special mask that fits over a _____.

84. To be effective, the mask must _____ to an individual's face.

QUESTIONS

Using what you have learned from the textbook, answer these questions.

85. Constant pressure from a nasal cannula may cause areas of irritation. What areas of the head and/or face may be irritated by the nasal cannula? _____

86. What type of lubricant should not be used on irritated areas of the nostrils? _____

87. a. A nasal cannula should be inspected frequently during use. What should the UAP check for when inspecting the prongs of a nasal cannula? _____

    b. What should the UAP do if she sees this material? _____

88. When a nasal cannula is not being used by an individual, what should the UAP do with the nasal cannula? _____

89. The flow rate for each method of oxygen delivery is different.

    a. What is the minimum liter flow rate for using a mask to deliver oxygen?

    b. What might happen if an individual uses a mask with a liter flow rate less than this?

90. How should a mask be worn for oxygen delivery? _____

91. a. When an individual is using a nonrebreathing mask, should the bag on the mask be inflated or deflated?

    b. When an individual is using a nonrebreathing mask, when should the UAP notify the individual's licensed health care provider that a problem may exist?

92. What is the maximum amount of time that an individual may use a nonrebreathing mask before he needs to be evaluated by his licensed health care provider?

93. Name four types of oxygen administration equipment.

a. _____

b. _____

c. _____

d. _____

94. What color are oxygen tanks in the United States? _____

95. What are the five differences between a liquid oxygen canister and an oxygen concentrator?

a. _____

b. _____

c. _____

d. _____

e. _____

96. When using liquid oxygen, what danger does the UAP have to be aware of?

_____

97. a. Liquid oxygen requires careful handling. If liquid oxygen touches the UAP's skin or clothing, what must the UAP do? _____

_____

b. Tanks and canisters of oxygen must be secured at all times. If a tank or canister of liquid oxygen falls or tips over, what must the UAP do?

_____

_____

_____

98. Briefly describe how an oxygen concentrator works. _____

_____

_____

_____

99. A mask is not used with an oxygen concentrator. Why not? _____

_____

100. When administering oxygen, a humidifier may be used. What is the benefit of using a humidifier when administering oxygen to an individual?

_____

_____

_____

101. A refillable humidifier bottle needs to be routinely cleaned and sterilized. How often should this be done? _____

102. A humidifier bottle must be filled with sterile, distilled water. Tap water should never be used. Why should the UAP never use tap water when filling a humidifier bottle?

_____
_____

103. When setting up a humidifier bottle, the UAP needs to routinely check the pressure relief valve. Briefly describe how to check the pressure relief valve.

_____
_____
_____
_____

104. When a humidifier bottle is being used in the administration of oxygen, how may the UAP tell that an individual is receiving the oxygen as ordered?

_____
_____

105. It is helpful to elevate the head of an individual's bed when she is receiving oxygen. Why is this so? _____
_____

106. There are times during the administration of oxygen when an individual will need to remove her mask and wear a nasal cannula for a period of time. Why might this be necessary? _____
_____
_____

107. Oxygen does not cause a fire, but it does support burning. For this reason, what six safety precautions must the UAP take when caring for an individual who uses oxygen?

   a. _____
   b. _____
   c. _____
   d. _____
   e. _____
   f. _____

COMPLETION

Complete the following statements by filling in the blanks.

108. List four basic respiratory positions.

   a. _____
   b. _____
   c. _____
   d. _____

109. List three steps for assisting an individual into high Fowler's position.

a. _____

b. _____

c. _____

110. In the _____ position, the individual sits up as straight as possible, leans slightly forward, and uses her forearms for support.

111. List four steps for assisting an individual into a tripod position.

a. _____

b. _____

c. _____

d. _____

112. Having the individual _____ on the side of the bed is another respiratory position.

113. The four respiratory positions allow the lungs to _____ and the airway to be kept _____.

114. List five symptoms of oxygen toxicity.

a. _____

b. _____

c. _____

d. _____

e. _____

115. If an individual receiving oxygen therapy reports any of the symptoms of oxygen toxicity, the UAP must immediately contact the _____.

116. An incentive spirometer may be used to prevent _____ and _____.

CLINICAL APPLICATIONS

Read the following paragraphs. Using what you have learned from the textbook, answer the questions.

Mrs. Caraballo has been diagnosed with congestive heart failure. She has a licensed HCP order for oxygen that reads O_2 @ 2 L/min via nasal cannula.

117. List the possible symptoms of oxygen toxicity.

a. _____

b. _____

c. _____

d. _____

e. _____

118. What should you tell Mrs. Caraballo's family and friends regarding safety measures while she is using her oxygen?

_____
_____

119. Your supervisor asks you to make some signs to alert people that Mrs. Caraballo is using oxygen. What would you write on the signs? Where would you put the signs?

_____
_____

A documentation sample for an individual using an incentive spirometer follows. Read the note. Answer the questions following the note.

On 11/17/09 an incentive spirometer is ordered for Mrs. Kline by her licensed health care provider at 8:30 a.m.

Mrs. Kline's progress note reads as follows:

11/17/09 8:40 AM Instructed in use of spirometer. Pointer set at 1000 cc. Assisted with use of incentive spirometer. R16 shallow and whistling. Productive cough with sm to mod amt of thick, greenish gray sputum. Total amt sputum approximately 4 cc. c/o mild dizziness after third inhalation. Refused further use of spirometer. Licensed HCP notified.

120. At what time did Mrs. Kline begin her use of the incentive spirometer? _____

_____
_____

121. What was the rate and description of Mrs. Kline's respirations before the use of her incentive spirometer?

_____

122. What was the lung volume on the incentive spirometer set at? _____

123. What was the description and amount of sputum Mrs. Kline expectorated? _____

_____
_____

124. Was any information left out of this progress note? _____

_____

QUESTIONS

Using what you have learned in the textbook, answer these questions.

125. Briefly describe sleep apnea. _____

_____
_____
_____

126. How does a CPAP device work? _____

127. When applying the CPAP face mask, why is it important to wash the individual's face first? _____

128. Why is it helpful to elevate the head of the individual's bed during use of a CPAP device? _____

CLINICAL APPLICATIONS

A documentation sample for an individual who uses a CPAP device follows. Read the note. Answer the questions following the note.

> On 4/19/10 Mrs. Salvo's licensed health care provider orders a CPAP device for her to use during sleep.
>
> Mrs. Salvo's progress note reads as follows:
>
> **4/19/10 10:00 PM CPAP applied**
>
> **4/20/10 6:45 AM CPAP removed. P 66 R 12. Appears well rested. States, "I've been sleeping pretty well with that thing on, believe it or not."**

129. At what time and on what date was Mrs. Salvo's CPAP device placed on her? _____

130. At what time was the CPAP device removed? _____

131. What were her initial respiratory rate and description? _____

132. What were her respiratory rate and pulse on removal of the CPAP device? _____

133. Was any information missing from the documentation? If so, what information was missing? _____

SUMMARY

Administration of oxygen is a procedure that requires a written licensed health care provider order. Oxygen is administered following the same guidelines as other medications. The UAP must use her skills of observation to monitor any changes or adverse reactions that an individual may have when using oxygen. This chapter provides the UAP with information regarding administration of oxygen, monitoring and reporting an individual's response to oxygen therapy, and guidelines for documentation of oxygen administration.

Chapter 9
Administration of Enemas

Learning Objectives

After completing the following exercises, you should be able to:

1. Spell and define terms.
2. List three reasons enemas are administered.
3. Describe three types of enemas.
4. List five types of enema solutions.
5. Describe a cleansing enema.
6. Describe a ready-to-use (prepackaged) enema.
7. Describe an oil retention enema.
8. Demonstrate the administration of a cleansing enema.
9. Demonstrate the administration of a ready-to-use (prepackaged) enema.
10. List seven guidelines for documenting the administration of an enema.

INTRODUCTION

The exercises you complete in this chapter address the following key concepts from the textbook chapter:

- medical reasons for administering an enema
- types of enemas and enema solutions
- procedures for administering various types of enemas
- documenting the administration of an enema

VOCABULARY

Define the following terms.

1. colon _____
2. endoscopy _____
   _____
3. feces _____
4. flatus _____
5. proctoscopy _____
   _____
6. rectum _____
7. sigmoidoscopy _____
   _____
8. constipation _____
9. enema _____
   _____

CHOICES

10. There are many different causes of constipation. In the following group of terms, circle each term that may be a cause of constipation.

    aging   high blood pressure   inactivity   relaxation   immobility
    diabetes   high cholesterol   exercise   walking   diet
    obesity   stress   medications   surgery   disease

COMPLETION

Complete the following statements by filling in the blanks.

11. List three reasons an enema may be administered.
    a. _____
    b. _____
    c. _____

12. List three reasons a rectal medication may be given.

a. _____

b. _____

c. _____

13. When preparing an individual for _____ tests, _____, or other procedures, enemas may be part of the preparation. The enema _____ the bowel. The licensed health care provider is then able to _____ on examination or during surgery.

14. List the three basic types of enemas.

a. _____

b. _____

c. _____

15. List five enema solutions.

a. _____

b. _____

c. _____

d. _____

e. _____

QUESTIONS

Using what you have learned from the textbook, answer these questions.

16. Give an example of a situation in which an individual's licensed health care provider would order a cleansing enema.

_____

_____

_____

17. Give an example of a situation in which an individual's licensed health care provider would order a ready-to-use (prepackaged) enema.

_____

_____

_____

18. Give an example of a situation in which an individual's licensed health care provider would order an oil retention enema. _____

_____

_____

19. Explain the meaning of a licensed health care provider order that reads, "Enemas until clear." _____

_____

_____

20. Most workplaces have guidelines stating the maximum number of cleansing enemas that an individual may be given at one time. If the UAP's workplace does not have such guidelines, what should the UAP do?

    _____
    _____
    _____

21. Ready-to-use (prepackaged) enemas are available in most grocery stores, pharmacies, and department stores. Before the UAP may administer a ready-to-use (prepackaged) enema to an individual, what is required?

    _____
    _____
    _____

22. Of the three types of enemas most commonly used, which type of enema is used primarily in an acute care setting? _____
    _____

23. When preparing to administer an enema to an individual, the UAP should help the individual into a position where she is lying on her left side with her left leg out straight and her right leg bent forward and up toward her stomach. Why is this position the most common position for an individual who is receiving an enema?

    _____
    _____
    _____

CHOICES

24. Read the following list of items. Circle each item that may be used in the administration of a cleansing enema.

    disposable enema kit
    towel or disposable pad
    trash bags
    clean paper toilet tissue
    water-soluble lubricating gel
    IV pole
    hot water bottle
    petroleum-based lubricating gel
    soap
    bed sheet
    bedside commode
    towel
    liquid enema solution
    basin
    paper towel
    syringe
    bedpan with cover
    disposable applicator
    gloves
    pillow
    ice

25. Read the following list of items. Circle each item that may be used in the administration of a ready-to-use (prepackaged) enema.

disposable enema kit

petroleum-based lubricating gel

trash bags

towel or disposable pad

water-soluble lubricating gel

hot water bottle

bedside commode

disposable prepackaged enema

soap

liquid enema solution

paper towel

syringe

bed sheet

clean paper toilet tissue

towel

pillow

ice

bedpan with cover

gloves

basin

warm water

ADMINISTRATION OF AN ENEMA

Whether the UAP is administering a cleansing enema or a ready-to-use (prepackaged) enema to an individual, there is a series of steps the UAP must complete. Although the methods for giving each type of enema differ, the steps leading up to the actual administration of the enema are the same.

26. Read the instructions below. Place them in the correct order by placing a number 1 next to the first step, a number 2 next to the second step, and so on. There are 17 steps total.

_____ Explain the procedure to the individual. Tell the individual that she may have a feeling of fullness or the need to move her bowels during administration of the enema. Instruct the individual to report any feelings of cramping or abdominal pain if they occur.

_____ Put on gloves.

_____ Wash hands.

_____ Cover the individual with a towel or blanket. Lower the individual's pants.

_____ Identify the individual to whom the enema is being given.

_____ Provide privacy.

_____ Encourage the individual to relax. Speak calmly. Playing soothing music may be helpful.

_____ Prepare the equipment in the utility room or the individual's bathroom.

_____ Place a disposable pad on the bed under the individual.

_____ Verify the licensed health care provider order.

_____ If possible, raise the bed to a comfortable and safe working height.

_____ Place a chair at the foot or at the side of the bed. Cover the chair with a disposable pad or towel. Place the equipment, including a bedpan if one will be used, on the covered chair.

_____ Take the equipment to the individual's bedside.

_____ Wash hands.

_____ Have the individual lie down on her left side, with her left leg out straight. Her right leg should be bent at the hip, with the knee bent forward and upward toward the stomach. If need be, assist the individual with positioning.

_____ Have the individual urinate, if possible, before giving the enema.

_____ Gather all the equipment needed.

CLINICAL APPLICATIONS

Read the following clinical scenarios. Using what you have learned from the textbook, answer the questions that follow each scenario.

Scenario #1: Mr. Sampson will be having a sigmoidoscopy tomorrow morning. Part of your assignment this evening is to help Mr. Sampson prepare for his upcoming procedure. Mr. Sampson's licensed HCP has ordered, "Cleansing enemas until clear."

27. Before you begin to prepare an enema for Mr. Sampson, there are three steps you must complete. What are those three steps? _____

28. What is the next step you must take as a UAP if the workplace guidelines are not specific regarding the maximum number of cleansing enemas that may be given?

29. List the equipment you will need to gather in order to give an enema to Mr. Sampson.

30. How would you prepare the cleansing enema for administration? _____

31. Write down what you would tell Mr. Sampson before administering his enema.

32. Explain the series of steps that must be completed before you can actually administer the enema to Mr. Sampson. _____

33. Explain the series of steps required to administer the enema to Mr. Sampson.

34. When you have administered approximately half of the enema solution, Mr. Sampson begins yelling, "Oh, it hurts! Oh, my stomach!" He begins sweating and grimacing. What should you do?

35. Write a progress note documenting what happened during administration of the enema to Mr. Sampson. Use today's date and the time of 7:30 p.m.

Scenario #2: You have been instructed to assist Mrs. Jefferson with self-administration of an enema to relieve constipation. Mrs. Jefferson's licensed health care provider has ordered a Fleet® enema. The enema solution is a ready-to-use, prepackaged enema.

36. It is now around 3 p.m. When would be a good time of day for Mrs. Jefferson to self-administer her enema?

37. What specific information do you need from the licensed HCP order to correctly assist Mrs. Jefferson to give herself the enema?

38. Write down what you would do to help Mrs. Jefferson prepare for self-administering her enema.

39. Mrs. Jefferson successfully self-administers the enema as ordered by her licensed HCP. Around 15 minutes after doing so, she requests your help in getting to the bathroom. What three things do you need to make sure of before you help Mrs. Jefferson?

    _____

    _____

40. What should you tell Mrs. Jefferson as you assist her to the bathroom?

    _____

    _____

41. Mrs. Jefferson successfully passes a moderate BM. Write a progress note documenting Mrs. Jefferson's self-administration of the Fleet® enema as ordered by her licensed HCP. Use today's date and the time of 8:45 p.m.

    _____

    _____

    _____

    _____

    _____

    _____

    _____

SUMMARY

In her role as caregiver, the UAP may be asked to administer an enema. It is important for the UAP to know her state regulations and workplace policies for enema administration. It is also important for the UAP to know proper and safe administration techniques and documentation guidelines. This chapter provides the UAP with information regarding types of enemas and solutions, administration of various types of enemas, and guidelines for documentation of enema administration.

Chapter 10
Care and Use of Gastrostomy and Jejunostomy Tubes

Learning Objectives
After completing the following exercises, you should be able to:
1. Spell and define terms.
2. Describe three types of feeding tubes.
3. Explain the differences between a nasogastric tube, a gastrostomy tube, and a jejunostomy tube.
4. Describe the difference between a continuous tube feeding and an intermittent tube feeding.
5. List four advantages of a continuous tube feeding.
6. Demonstrate the administration of a continuous tube feeding.
7. Describe the difference between the bolus method and the gravity drip method.
8. List two advantages and two disadvantages of an intermittent tube feeding.
9. Demonstrate the administration of an intermittent tube feeding by bolus.
10. Demonstrate the administration of an intermittent tube feeding by the gravity drip method.
11. List three contraindications for a tube feeding.
12. Demonstrate the care of gastrostomy and jejunostomy tubes.
13. Demonstrate the procedure for flushing gastrostomy and jejunostomy tubes.
14. Demonstrate the procedure for checking for residual feeding.
15. List six basic guidelines for caring for gastrostomy and jejunostomy equipment.
16. List ten guidelines to follow when caring for an individual with a gastrostomy or jejunostomy tube.
17. Demonstrate the administration of medication via gastrostomy and jejunostomy tube when the individual is receiving a continuous tube feeding.
18. Demonstrate the administration of medication via gastrostomy and jejunostomy tube when the individual is receiving an intermittent tube feeding.

INTRODUCTION

The exercises you complete in this chapter address the following key concepts from the textbook chapter:

- appropriate use of a nasogastric tube, a gastrostomy tube, and a jejunostomy tube
- differences among methods of feeding, and advantages of each
- care of a gastrostomy tube and a jejunostomy tube and the related equipment
- care of an individual who has a feeding tube in place
- administration of medication using various types of feeding tubes and various methods of feeding

VOCABULARY

Define the following terms.

1. aspiration _____
2. incision _____
3. navel _____
4. sternum _____
5. jejunum _____
6. bolus _____

COMPLETION

Complete the following statements by filling in the blanks.

7. A nasogastric (NG) tube is inserted through the _____ into the _____.

8. A gastrostomy tube (G-tube) is inserted into an individual's _____ _____ through a _____.

9. A jejunostomy tube (J-tube) is inserted into an individual's _____ through a _____.

10. Once the NG tube, G-tube, or J-tube is inserted, an _____ is taken to see if the tube is _____.

QUESTIONS

Using what you have learned from the textbook, answer these questions.

11. Of the three types of feeding tubes—nasogastric, gastrostomy, and jejunostomy tubes—which type is the easiest to dislodge? _____

12. Why is the dislodging of this tube such a problem? _____

13. What are the differences between a gastrostomy tube and a jejunostomy tube? _____

14. What is a PEG tube? _____

15. Why is a PEG tube commonly used when an individual needs a feeding tube? _____

16. There are two different types of tube feedings, a continuous tube feeding and an intermittent tube feeding. What are the differences between the two feedings? _____

17. What are the differences between a bolus feeding and a gravity drip feeding? _____

18. Regardless of the feeding method, there are two important details that the UAP must check before he administers a tube feeding. What are these two details?

    a. _____
    b. _____

19. Why are these details important? _____

20. What information is contained in the written licensed health care provider order for a tube feeding? _____

_____

_____

21. Describe the Fowler's position. _____

_____

_____

22. Regardless of the feeding method used, when administering the formula it is important that the feeding tube never be completely empty. Why is this important?

_____

_____

_____

CLINICAL APPLICATIONS

Read the written licensed health care provider orders for tube feeding formulas that follow. Answer the questions after each order. Remember that 30 mL = 1 ounce.

23. Order reads: *1/4 strength Enfamil 12 mL via jejunostomy tube qh for 10 hours*

    Available: Enfamil 3-ounce bottles.

    a. How would you mix the formula as ordered? _____

    _____

    b. How much liquid will be given in total? _____

    c. How many bottles of Enfamil will you need to open? _____

    d. How much Enfamil will be left? _____

24. Order reads: *3/4 strength Sustacal 360 mL over 4 hours via gastrostomy tube*

    Available: Sustacal 10-ounce cans.

    a. How would you mix the formula as ordered? _____

    _____

    b. How much liquid will be given in total? _____

    c. How many cans of Sustacal will you need to open? _____

    d. How much Sustacal will be left? _____

25. Order reads: *2/3 strength Ensure. Give 90 mL qh for 5 hours via jejunostomy tube*

    Available: Ensure 8-ounce cans.

    a. How would you mix the formula as ordered? _____

    _____

    b. How much liquid will be given in total? _____

    c. How many cans of Ensure will you need to open? _____

    d. How much Ensure will be left? _____

26. Order reads: *1/8 strength Ensure. Give 160 mL stat via jejunostomy tube*

Available: Ensure 4-ounce cans.

   a. How would you mix the formula as ordered? _____

   _____

   b. How much liquid will be given in total? _____

   c. How many cans of Ensure will you need to open? _____

   d. How much Ensure will be left? _____

27. Order reads: *1/2 strength Ensure 55 mL hourly for 10 hours via gastrostomy tube*

Available: Ensure 12-ounce cans.

   a. How would you mix the formula as ordered? _____

   _____

   b. How much liquid will be given in total? _____

   c. How many cans of Ensure will you need to open? _____

   d. How much Ensure will be left? _____

CHOICES

28. From the choices below, circle each piece of equipment that is used when giving a continuous or intermittent tube feeding.

formula	formula bag	emesis basin	sterile gauze pads
paper towel	clean washcloth	mild soap	warm water
hypoallergenic one-inch tape	60 mL (cc) syringe	cotton swabs	sterile gloves
	nonsterile gloves	towel	medication

29. From the choices below, circle each piece of equipment that is used when caring for a gastrostomy or jejunostomy tube with a dressing and an incision site that has not healed.

formula	formula bag	emesis basin	sterile gauze pads
paper towel	clean washcloth	mild soap	warm water
hypoallergenic one-inch tape	60 mL (cc) syringe	cotton swabs	sterile gloves
	nonsterile gloves	towel	medication

30. From the choices below, circle each piece of equipment that is used when flushing a gastrostomy or jejunostomy tube.

formula	formula bag	emesis basin	sterile gauze pads
paper towel	clean washcloth	mild soap	warm water
hypoallergenic one-inch tape	60 mL (cc) syringe	cotton swabs	sterile gloves
	nonsterile gloves	towel	medication

31. From the choices below, circle each piece of equipment that is used when checking for residual feeding.

formula	formula bag	emesis basin	sterile gauze pads
paper towel	clean washcloth	mild soap	warm water
hypoallergenic one-inch tape	60 mL (cc) syringe	cotton swabs	sterile gloves
	nonsterile gloves	towel	medication

32. From the choices below, circle each piece of equipment that is used when giving medication through a gastrostomy or jejunostomy tube.

formula	formula bag	emesis basin	sterile gauze pads
paper towel	clean washcloth	mild soap	warm water
hypoallergenic one-inch tape	60 mL (cc) syringe	cotton swabs	sterile gloves
	nonsterile gloves	towel	medication

COMPLETION

Complete the following statements by filling in the blanks.

33. The word "contraindicated" means _____ .

34. List four conditions in which tube feeding is contraindicated.

a. _____

b. _____

c. _____

d. _____

MATCHING

Draw lines to connect each term in the left column with its definition in the right column.

35. diffuse peritonitis   a. abnormal pathways from the intestines to the skin

36. paralytic ileus   b. decreased blood supply to the gastrointestinal system

37. pancreatitis

38. enterocutaneous fistulae   c. the slowing or absence of intestinal peristalsis

39. GI ischemia   d. widespread inflammation of the lining of the abdominal cavity

     e. inflammation of the pancreas

CLINICAL APPLICATIONS

Read each of the following scenarios. After reading each scenario, write a note to document the event. If the situation requires a call to the licensed health care provider and/or workplace supervisor, presume that you have made those calls and are waiting to hear from the licensed HCP and/or supervisor. Use today's date.

40. Part of your assignment today is to administer a continuous tube feeding to Gerald, who has a gastrostomy tube. The written licensed health care provider order reads:

1/2 strength Sustacal 720 mL over 8 hours via gastrostomy tube.

You are able to give Gerald the entire feeding without incident.

41. Your assignment today includes administering a bolus feeding to Suzanne. The written licensed health care provider order reads:

1/4 strength Ensure 300 mL bolus via gastrostomy tube.

After you administer the bolus feeding, you notice that Suzanne's abdomen is bloated and she is complaining of nausea.

42. Part of your assignment today is to care for Carl's jejunostomy tube site. This is a new J-tube. There is still a dressing over the incision. When you remove the dressing to give care, you smell a foul odor. You observe redness and thick, yellow-green drainage around the site. You also notice a space of approximately one inch between Carl's abdominal wall and the length marker on his J-tube.

43. Your assignment today includes flushing Roberta's gastrostomy tube. You use 50 mL (cc) of water to flush her tube. You complete the procedure without incident.

_____
_____
_____
_____
_____
_____
_____
_____

44. Part of your assignment today is to check David's gastrostomy tube for residual feeding. You notice some swelling around the tube site. During the check, you use 50 mL (cc) to flush the tube. You remove a total of 150 mL (cc) of fluid from David's stomach.

_____
_____
_____
_____
_____
_____
_____
_____

45. Your assignment today includes administering Dilantin to Paul. Paul has a J-tube. He receives a continuous feeding. The written licensed health care provider order reads:

phenytoin (Dilantin) 125 mg/5 mL oral suspension 250 mg via jejunostomy tube tid.

After you administer the medication, you leave the tube feeding off. Paul remains in the Fowler's position. You leave the room to care for other individuals. You are gone for around 60 minutes. When you come back to restart his feeding pump, Paul is no longer in Fowler's position. The head of Paul's bed is flat. You notice that the tube feeding is running. Paul's skin is pale, cool, and clammy. His breathing is irregular and gurgling. You immediately raise the head of his bed and call for help. You ask the staff member who arrives to call 911 and Paul's licensed HCP immediately.

_____
_____
_____
_____
_____

46. Part of your assignment includes administering ibuprofen to Angela. Angela has a gastrostomy tube with an intermittent feeding. The written licensed health care provider order reads:

> *ibuprofen (Motrin) 200 mg 1 tab every 6 hours prn via gastrostomy tube for menstrual cramps. Tablet may be crushed for administration via gastrostomy tube.*

You are able to administer the medication without incident. Presume that you have already documented on the medication sheet.

SUMMARY

In his daily assignment, the UAP may be asked to administer feedings and medications through a gastrostomy, jejunostomy, or PEG tube. Following the correct procedures, communicating clearly, and asking for additional information and assistance will all help the UAP to perform these tasks safely and effectively. Remember, if there is any doubt or uncertainty, the UAP should contact his supervisor and the individual's licensed health care provider before proceeding with any task involving a gastrostomy, jejunostomy, or PEG tube. Doing so will help the UAP to complete his tasks in the best and safest way possible.

Chapter 11
Administration of Epinephrine by EpiPen

Learning Objectives

After completing the following exercises, you should be able to:

1. Spell and define terms.
2. List five causes of anaphylaxis.
3. List five initial signs and symptoms of anaphylaxis.
4. List four life-threatening signs and symptoms of anaphylaxis.
5. Explain why anaphylaxis is life threatening.
6. List four items that must be included in the licensed health care provider order for the administration of epinephrine.
7. List three possible side effects of epinephrine.
8. List two classes of medications that may interact with epinephrine.
9. Describe five requirements for the proper storage and handling of epinephrine.
10. Describe the emergency procedure to be followed when epinephrine is administered.
11. Demonstrate the use of an EpiPen Auto-Injector.

INTRODUCTION

The exercises you complete in this chapter address the following key concepts from the textbook chapter:

- causes, signs, and symptoms of anaphylaxis
- licensed health care provider order for administration of epinephrine
- side effects of epinephrine
- medication interactions with epinephrine
- administration, storage, and handling of an EpiPen
- emergency procedures for administration of an EpiPen

VOCABULARY

Define the following terms.

1. anaphylaxis _____

_____

2. allergen _____
3. hives _____
4. bronchodilator _____

_____

QUESTIONS

Using what you have learned from the textbook, answer these questions.

5. What is anaphylaxis? _____

_____

6. Why does anaphylaxis occur? _____

_____

_____

7. Why is anaphylaxis life threatening? _____

_____

_____

COMPLETION

Complete the following statements by filling in the blanks.

8. The most common cause of anaphylaxis is _____ .
9. Individuals most likely to have an anaphylactic reaction to penicillin receive the penicillin by the _____ route or for _____ therapy.

104 Module 3 Medication Administration

10. List four other causes of anaphylaxis.

    a. _____
    b. _____
    c. _____
    d. _____

11. An anaphylactic reaction may happen in _____ or up to _____ after exposure to the allergen.

12. List six initial signs and symptoms of anaphylaxis.

    a. _____
    b. _____
    c. _____
    d. _____
    e. _____
    f. _____

13. List four life-threatening signs and symptoms of anaphylaxis.

    a. _____
    b. _____
    c. _____
    d. _____

14. Because death may result in only a few minutes, the UAP must always know the _____ and _____ _____ that the individuals in her care may have.

QUESTIONS

Using what you have learned from the textbook, answer these questions.

15. What is the preferred medication for the treatment of anaphylaxis? _____
    _____

16. What type of medication is this? _____
    _____

17. Briefly describe three ways in which this medication works.

    a. _____
    b. _____
    c. _____

18. An EpiPen Auto-Injector is available in two strengths. List the two strengths that the EpiPen Auto-Injector comes in.

    a. _____
    b. _____

19. What are four specific pieces of information that must be included in a licensed health care provider order for an EpiPen?

   a. _____
   b. _____
   c. _____
   d. _____

20. Why is it important for the UAP to have a licensed health care provider order to carry an EpiPen?

   _____
   _____
   _____

21. It is important for the individual at risk for anaphylaxis or her UAP to always carry an EpiPen. In addition, EpiPens should always be kept in other easily accessible places. Where are three other places EpiPens should be kept?

   a. _____
   b. _____
   c. _____

22. The storage and handling of EpiPens are similar to the storage and handling of other syringes. EpiPens, for example, must be accounted for on a routine basis. How are EpiPens accounted for at the UAP's workplace? _____
   _____
   _____
   _____

COMPLETION

Complete the following statements.

23. List three common side effects of epinephrine.

   a. _____
   b. _____
   c. _____

24. Many medications may interact with epinephrine. List three types of medication that may interact with epinephrine.

   a. _____
   b. _____
   c. _____

25. Because of possible medication interactions, what must the UAP do immediately after administering an EpiPen? _____
   _____

26. An EpiPen may be administered at only one specific site. What site must be used for the administration of an EpiPen? How is an EpiPen administered?

_____
_____
_____

CLINICAL SCENARIO

Read the following clinical scenario. Answer the questions.

Your day program is having a party to celebrate birthdays for the month. There are cookies, cakes, and pastries on the table. One of the individuals you supervise, Jennifer, has an allergy to nuts. She is usually able to make good dietary choices, but at parties she tends to need supervision to avoid foods that may contain nuts. When you enter the room, you see Jennifer at the table. She is already chewing something. In about 15 seconds, she turns to you. You notice changes in her appearance. Her skin is flushed. Her lips are swollen. She is clutching her abdomen. She says to you, "I feel terrible. My stomach is killing me!" She vomits.

27. What is happening to Jennifer? _____
_____

28. How do you know this? _____
_____

29. What must you do immediately? _____
_____

30. What do you do next? _____
_____

31. You accompany Jennifer to the emergency room. What do you need to tell the health care professionals at the emergency room? _____
_____

32. What do you do last? _____

33. Write a progress note documenting the event. Use today's date and a time of 2:30 p.m. If this situation requires a call to Jennifer's licensed health care provider and/or the workplace supervisor, presume that you have made those calls and are waiting for any return calls as appropriate.

_____
_____
_____
_____
_____
_____
_____
_____

SUMMARY

Anaphylaxis, a severe allergic reaction, is a life-threatening emergency. It is imperative that the UAP know the allergy and reaction history of the individuals she cares for. It is also extremely important that the UAP know the emergency procedures for treating anaphylaxis and can react quickly in such a situation. The UAP not only gives care to individuals but also helps to keep them safe. Understanding what to do in an emergency such as anaphylaxis will help the UAP give the best care she can to the individuals she works with.

MODULE 4
MEDICATIONS AND THEIR EFFECTS ON THE BODY

Chapter 12
Body Organizations and Systems

Learning Objectives

After completing the exercises in this chapter, you should be able to:

1. Spell and define terms.
2. Understand the organization of the body, from cell level to cavities and organs.
3. Understand each body system as it pertains to medication administration.
4. Describe three common disorders of each body system.

INTRODUCTION

The exercises you complete in this chapter will address the following key concepts from the textbook chapter:

- organization of the human body
- systems of the body
- common disorders of each body system

VOCABULARY

Define the following terms.

1. cell _____
2. tissue _____
3. organ _____
4. membrane _____
5. cavities _____
6. system _____

COMPLETION

Complete the following statements by filling in the blanks.

7. All parts of the body work together, meaning they are _____.

8. The _____ is the basic unit of the body.

9. Groups of similar cells are organized into _____.

10. Different tissues form _____.

11. The organs are organized into _____, which perform _____.

MATCHING

Draw lines to connect each term in the left column with its definition in the right column.

12. epithelial cells
13. nerve cells
14. muscle cells
15. connective tissue
16. epithelial tissue
17. nervous tissue

a. present throughout the body to support and connect body parts
b. forms blood, bone, ligaments, and tendons
c. can absorb and produce fluids, eliminate waste, and protect structures in the body
d. forms the walls of body organs and cells
e. forms the walls of the heart
f. form protective coverings, sometimes make body fluids

18. skeletal muscle
19. cardiac muscle
20. smooth muscle
21. connective tissue

g. can shorten or lengthen to help move parts of the body

h. forms the brain, spinal cord, and nerves throughout the body; also found in sensory organs like eyes, ears, and taste buds

i. attached to bone for movement

j. carry electrical impulses that help us move, breathe, and use our senses

COMPLETION

Complete the following statements by filling in the blanks.

22. Organs perform specific activities that help the body to work as a whole. List seven major organs of the human body.

    a. _____
    b. _____
    c. _____
    d. _____
    e. _____
    f. _____
    g. _____

23. Membranes have three jobs. They _____, _____, and _____.

24. Mucous membranes produce a fluid called _____. They line body cavities that _____, such as the nose and throat.

25. Synovial membranes produce a fluid called _____, which reduces _____ in _____ movement. Synovial membranes line _____.

DIAGRAM

26. Following is a side view of the body cavities. Label each cavity from the list of choices under the diagram.

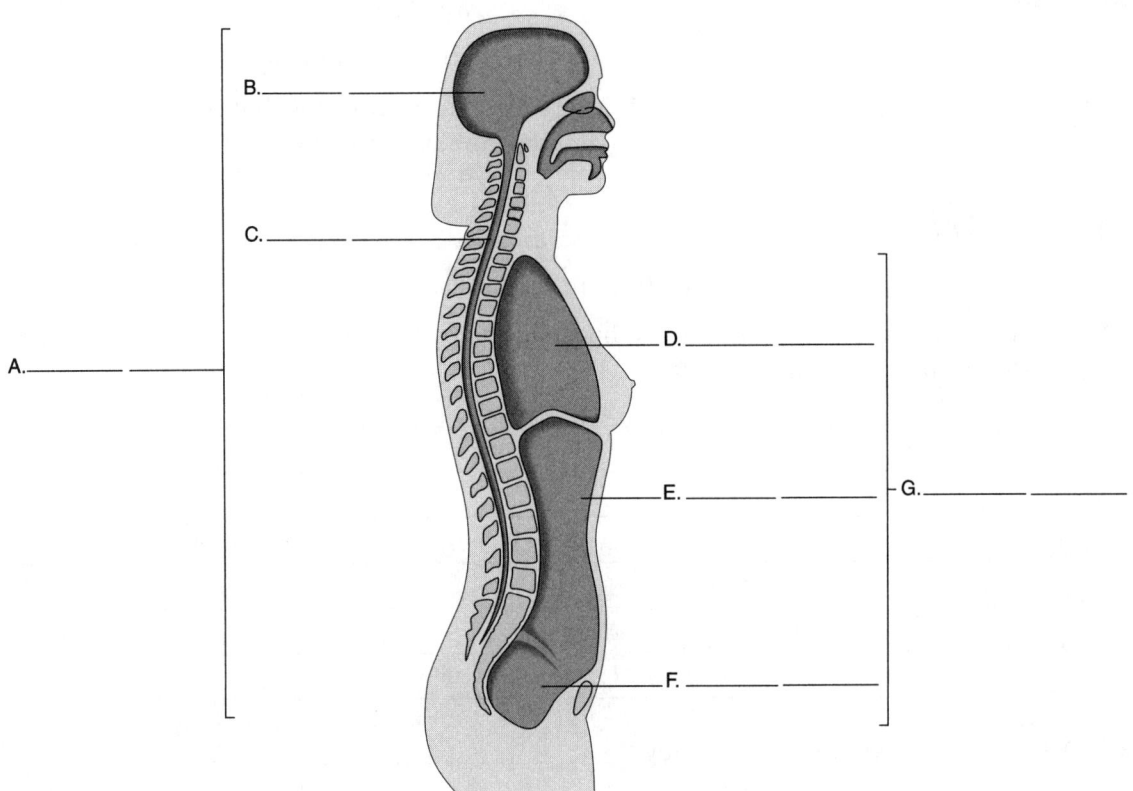

Figure 12-1 Side view of the body cavities *(Delmar/Cengage Learning)*

dorsal cavity   thoracic cavity   cranial cavity
pelvic cavity   ventral cavity   abdominal cavity
spinal cavity

QUESTIONS

Using what you have learned from the textbook, answer each question with one or two phrases or short sentences.

27. What are the functions of the cardiovascular, or circulatory, system?

_____

28. What organ drives the cardiovascular system?

_____

29. What do the blood vessels do? _____

30. In what direction do arteries carry blood? _____

_____

31. In what direction do veins carry blood? _____

_____

32. Briefly explain what each of the following structures do:
   a. capillaries _____
   b. lymphatic vessels _____
   c. lymph nodes _____
   d. spleen _____

DIAGRAM

33. The heart has four chambers. Below is a diagram of the heart. Label each of the chambers from the list of choices under the diagram.

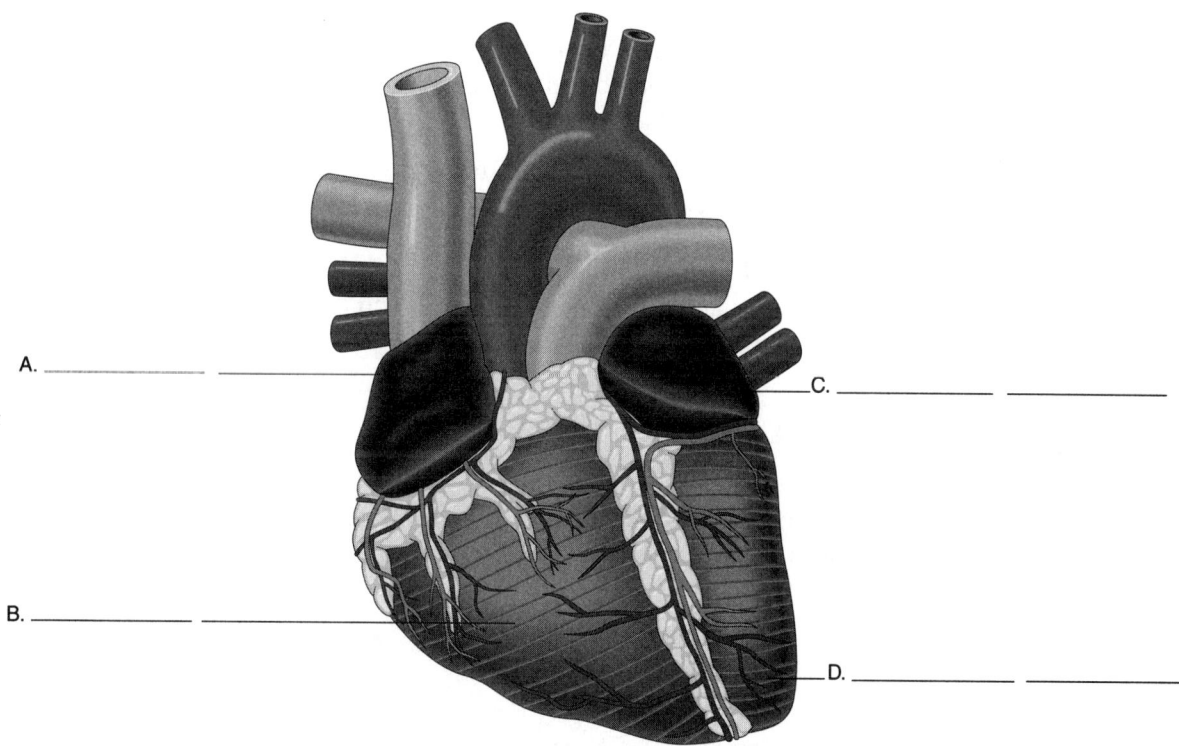

A. _____
B. _____
C. _____
D. _____

Figure 12-2 A diagram of the heart *(Delmar/Cengage Learning)*

right atrium   right ventricle   left atrium   left ventricle

COMPLETION

Complete the following statements by filling in the blanks.

34. Varicose veins and hypertension are two examples of diseases of the _____.

35. Congestive heart failure is one example of diseases of the _____.

36. Anemia and leukemia are examples of blood abnormalities. They are also called _____.

37. The endocrine system is made up of glands that release _____ or chemicals that control the body's activities and growth.

116   Module 4   Medications and Their Effects on the Body

38. List four common disorders of the endocrine system.
   a. _____
   b. _____
   c. _____
   d. _____

MATCHING

Draw lines to connect each term in the left column with its definition in the right column.

39. pituitary gland
40. pineal body
41. adrenal glands
42. gonads
43. thyroid gland
44. parathyroid gland
45. islets of Langerhans

a. produce insulin and glucagon, which control blood sugar
b. produces parathormone, which helps control the body's use of calcium and phosphorus
c. releases thyroxine, which controls metabolism, and thyrocalcitonin, which controls calcium and phosphorus levels
d. thought to be related to sexual growth
e. the "master gland" that controls most of the other glands
f. produce adrenalin and noradrenaline, elevate blood sugar levels, control sodium and potassium levels, produce cortisone, influence sex hormones
g. ovaries and testes

DIAGRAM

46. Below is a diagram of the gastrointestinal system. Label each structure from the list of choices under the diagram.

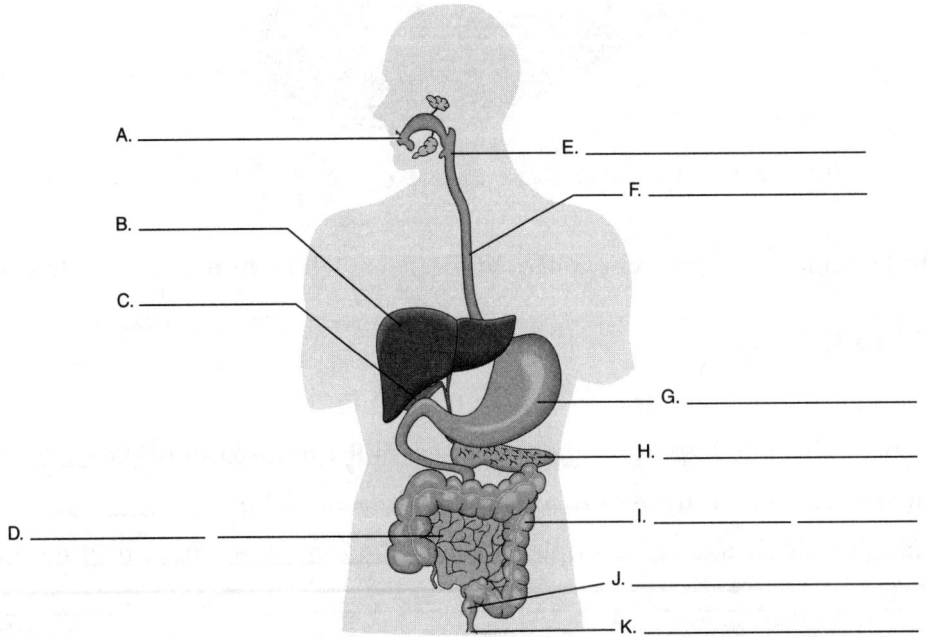

A. _____
B. _____
C. _____
D. _____
E. _____
F. _____
G. _____
H. _____
I. _____
J. _____
K. _____

Figure 12-3 Diagram of the gastrointestinal system *(Delmar/Cengage Learning)*

mouth	liver	anus	small intestine
large intestine	stomach	pharynx	rectum
esophagus	pancreas	gallbladder	

COMPLETION

Complete the following statements by filling in the blanks.

47. The gastrointestinal system is also called the _____ or _____.

48. The gastrointestinal system helps the body to _____, _____, and _____ nutrients, as well as to _____ waste.

49. A common disorder of the GI tract is cancer, also called _____.

50. Sores that are common in the colon, stomach, and duodenum are also called _____.

51. A hernia occurs when a structure pushes through a weakened area in a _____ that usually holds it in place.

52. A hernia in the groin is called an _____ hernia.

53. A hernia near the umbilicus or belly button is called an _____ hernia.

54. A hernia through a poorly healed incision is called an _____ hernia.

55. A hernia through the diaphragm is called a _____ hernia.

56. Another name for inflammation of the gallbladder is _____.

57. Another name for gallstones is _____.

58. Three GI disorders that happen in the large intestine and rectum are _____, _____, and _____.

QUESTIONS

Using what you have learned from the textbook, answer each question with one or two phrases or short sentences.

59. There are six structures in the integumentary system. What are the names of the structures in the integumentary system?

a. _____

b. _____

c. _____

d. _____

e. _____

f. _____

60. The skin is the largest organ in the body. What are the three jobs of the skin?

a. _____

b. _____

c. _____

61. a. What are the two layers of the skin? _____

b. What is contained in the top layer? _____

c. What is contained in the lower layer? _____

_____

62. How would skin tell us that someone:

a. has a fever? _____

b. has a low oxygen content in his blood? _____

c. has any type of acute illness? _____

d. has been doing strenuous activity? _____

63. What is the definition of a skin lesion? _____

_____

MATCHING

Draw lines to connect each term in the left column with its definition in the right column.

64. papules
65. vesicles
66. wheals
67. excoriation
68. abrasion
69. ecchymosis
70. laceration
71. pressure ulcers
72. decubitus ulcers
73. shearing
74. friction

a. the skin moves in one direction, and the structures under the skin move in the opposite direction

b. open areas of skin over a bony area

c. another name for pressure ulcers

d. a bruise

e. blisters

f. the skin rubs against another surface, even another area of skin

g. part of the skin has been scratched or scraped away

h. a scrape on the skin

i. a solid, raised, red area on the skin

j. hives

k. a cut, a break in the skin

CHOICES

75. From the list below, circle the body structures that are in the musculoskeletal system.

skeletal muscles	kidneys	brain	bones
spinal cord	blood vessels	lungs	heart
joints	nerves	ligaments	tendons

COMPLETION

Complete the statements below by filling in the blanks.

76. There are a total of _____,_____ bones in the human body and over _____ muscles in the human body.

77. Bones are solid structures made of _____, _____, and _____.

78. Bones are filled with marrow, which helps to produce _____.

79. Joints are places where _____ and where there might be _____.

80. Ligaments are _____, like rubber bands, that help to _____ the joints and _____ at these joints.

81. A small sac called a _____ holds fluid that surrounds the joint to help keep it _____.

82. Another name for skeletal muscles is _____ muscles.

83. Muscles can only shorten, or _____, and lengthen, or _____.

84. Strong fibers called _____ attach muscles to bones.

85. As muscles are used, they _____ strength. If muscles are not used, they _____ strength.

MATCHING

Draw lines to connect each term in the left column with its definition in the right column.

86. bursitis
87. arthritis
88. rheumatoid
89. osteoarthritis
90. gout
91. osteoporosis
92. fibromyalgia
93. fracture
94. total joint
95. amputation

a. a metabolic disease in which bones lose their mass and become very spongy, with very high risk for fracture

b. a joint is surgically removed and an artificial one is inserted

c. the surgical removal of a limb such as an arm arthritis

d. an inflammation of the bursa sac around a joint

e. any break in any bone

f. a chronic pain syndrome

g. a type of arthritis that affects the joint tissue and lining

h. a metabolic disease most common in the feet and legs

i. a type of arthritis that affects the cartilage in replacement between the bones that form a joint

j. an inflammation of the joints

DIAGRAM

96. Below are diagrams of a nerve cell. Label each structure from the list of choices under the diagram.

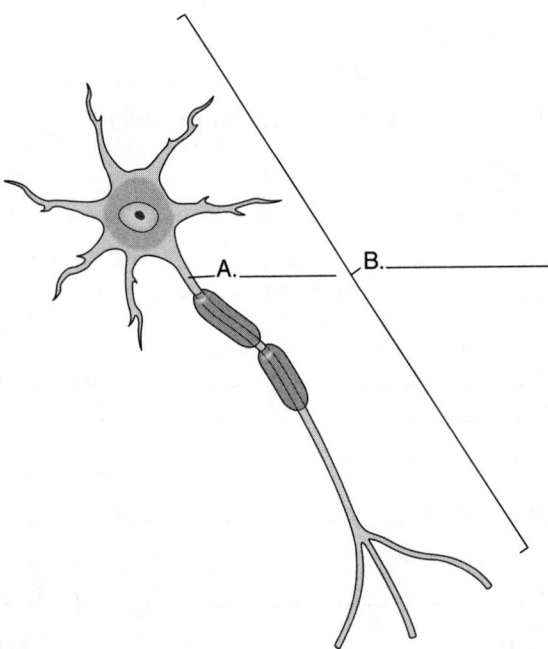

Figure 12-4a Diagram of a nerve cell *(Delmar/Cengage Learning)*

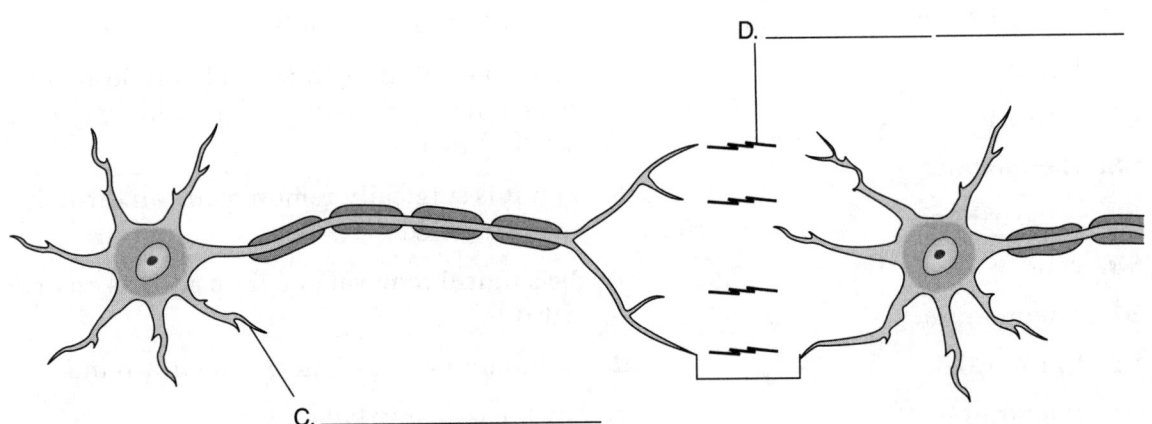

Figure 12-4b Diagram of a nerve cell *(Delmar/Cengage Learning)*

neuron   axon   dendrites   neurotransmitters

QUESTIONS

Using what you have learned from the textbook, answer each question with one or two phrases or short sentences.

97. What are the 10 structures that make up the nervous system?

a. _____
b. _____
c. _____
d. _____
e. _____
f. _____
g. _____
h. _____
i. _____
j. _____

98. What does the nervous system do? _____
_____

99. a. What are the two major components of the nervous system?
_____

b. What structures does the first component contain? _____
_____

c. What does the second component do? _____
_____

100. The brain is the powerhouse of the nervous system. List the three jobs that the brain does.

a. _____
b. _____
c. _____
_____
_____
_____

101. What does the spinal cord do? _____
_____

102. What do the sensory receptors do? _____
_____

103. The eye is a more highly developed sensory receptor. What are the two main actions of the eye?

a. _____
b. _____

104. The ear is another more highly developed sensory organ. What are the two main actions of the ear?

   a. _____

   b. _____

MATCHING

Draw lines to connect each term in the left column with its definition in the right column.

105. transient ischemic attack
106. cerebrovascular accident
107. aphasia
108. Parkinson's disease
109. multiple sclerosis
110. amyotropic lateral sclerosis
111. epilepsy
112. macular degeneration
113. otitis media
114. otosclerosis

a. a nervous disorder caused by a loss of myelin around central nervous system fibers

b. Lou Gehrig's disease, a progressive disease that causes muscle weakness and paralysis and is almost always fatal

c. a breakdown of the retina inside the eye, which causes loss of central vision

d. a progressive form of deafness

e. a stroke, caused by complete or partial loss of blood flow to the brain

f. a nervous disorder that causes tremors, muscle rigidity, and difficulty with voluntary movement

g. difficulty expressing or understanding communication or language

h. temporary decrease in blood flow to the brain, causing symptoms similar to a stroke that are temporary and reversible

i. an infection of the middle ear

j. a seizure disorder caused by recurring and temporary episodes of disrupted brain function

DIAGRAMS

115. Below is a diagram of the male reproductive system. Label each structure from the list of choices under the diagram.

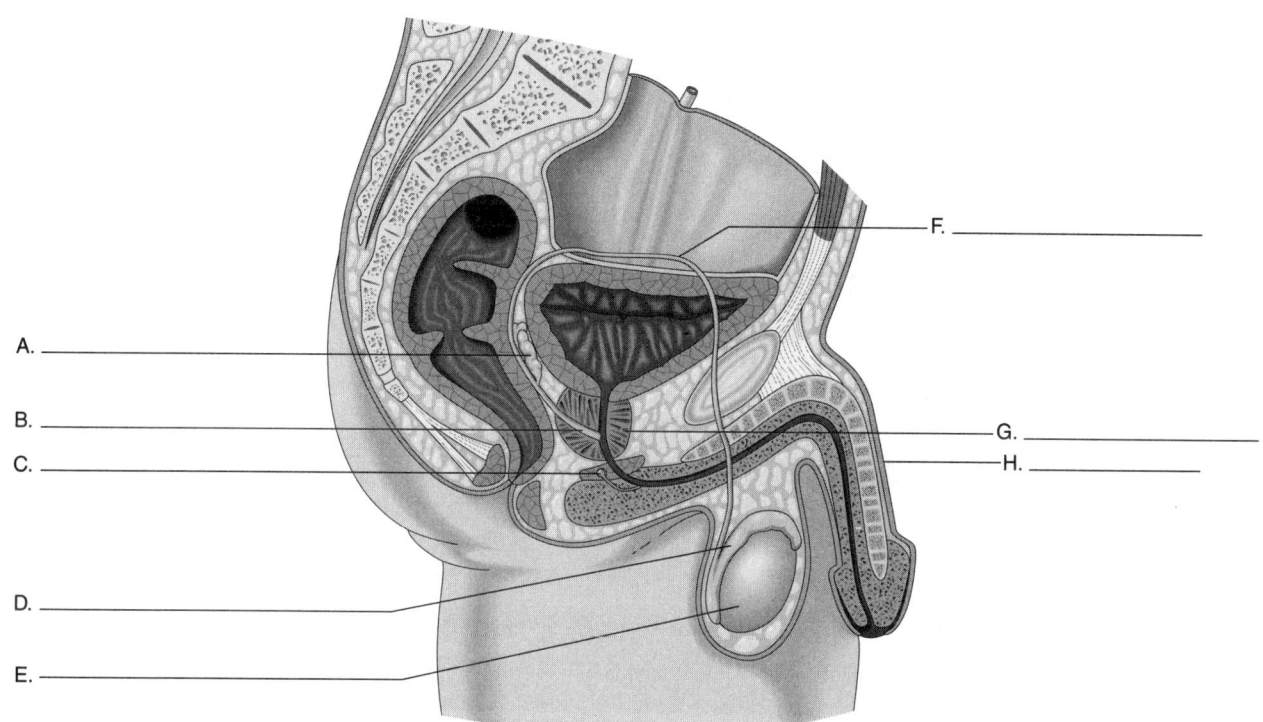

Figure 12-5 Diagram of the male reproductive system *(Delmar/Cengage Learning)*

| testes | seminal vesicles | Cowper's glands | vas deferens |
| epididymis | ejaculatory duct | penis | prostate gland |

124 Module 4 Medications and Their Effects on the Body

116. Below is a diagram of the female reproductive system. Label each structure from the list of choices under the diagram.

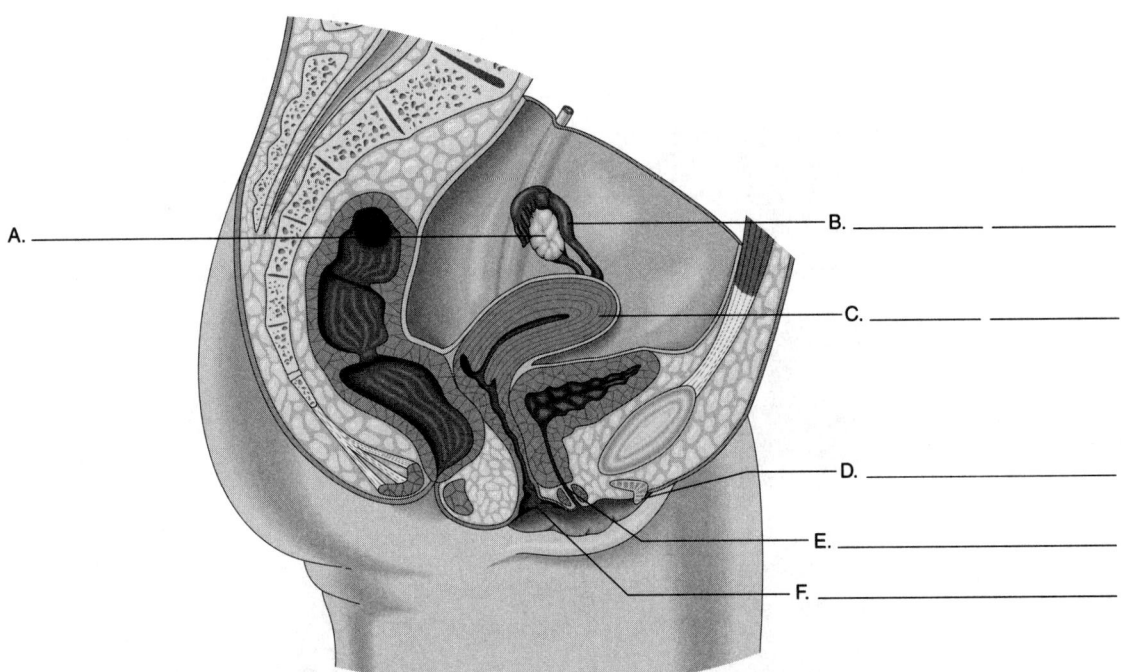

Figure 12-6 Diagram of the female reproductive system *(Delmar/Cengage Learning)*

urethra   ovary   uterus
clitoris   fallopian tubes vagina

COMPLETION

Complete the following statements by filling in the blanks.

117. The reproductive system is present in males and females. Both systems do two things. The systems produce _____ cells. They also produce _____ that control _____ characteristics.

118. The male reproductive system produces _____ and the hormone _____.

119. List two common disorders of the male reproductive system.
    a. _____
    b. _____

120. The female reproductive system triggers the process of _____ and _____ beginning at puberty.

121. The monthly cycle in which the ovum or egg is released into the uterus for possible fertilization is called _____.

122. If the egg is not fertilized, it is flushed from the uterus along with the lining of the uterus. This is called _____.

123. When the last ova are released from the ovaries, a stage called _____ is triggered.

124. List six common disorders of the female reproductive system.

   a. _____
   b. _____
   c. _____
   d. _____
   e. _____
   f. _____

125. List seven common sexually transmitted diseases and their causes.

   a. _____
   b. _____
   c. _____
   d. _____
   e. _____
   f. _____
   g. _____

DIAGRAM

126. Below is a diagram of the respiratory system. Label each structure from the list of choices under the diagram.

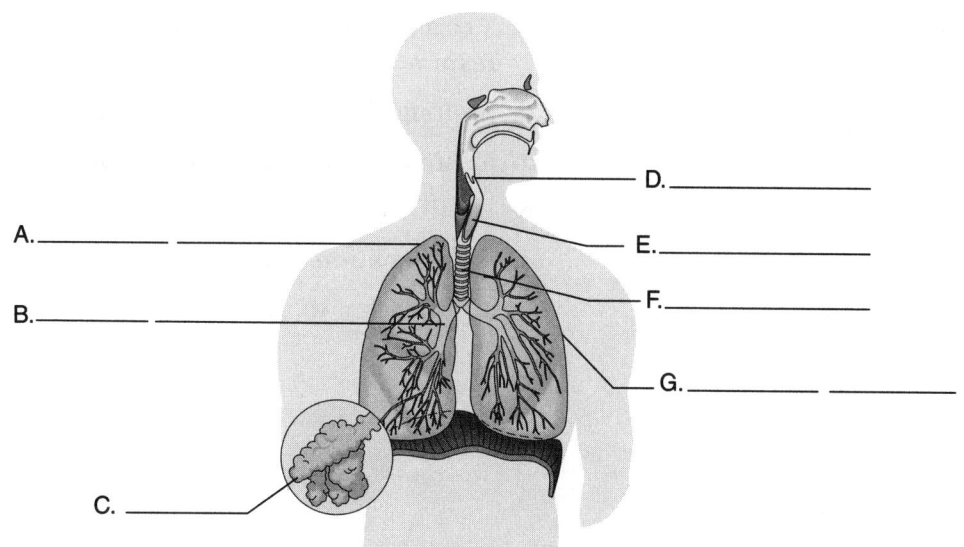

Figure 12-7 Diagram of the respiratory system *(Delmar/Cengage Learning)*

| pharynx | larynx | trachea | right bronchus |
| right lung | left lung | alveoli | |

QUESTIONS

Using what you have learned from the textbook, answer each question with one or two phrases or short sentences.

127. What five structures does air pass through as it goes to the lungs?

   a. _____
   b. _____
   c. _____
   d. _____
   e. _____

128. Describe what happens to air after it enters the lungs.

   _____
   _____
   _____

129. How does the respiratory system play a part in voice production? _____

   _____
   _____
   _____

MATCHING

Draw lines to connect each term in the left column with its definition in the right column.

130. hypoxemia
131. upper respiratory infection
132. pneumonia
133. chronic obstructive pulmonary disease
134. chronic bronchitis
135. emphysema
136. tracheostomy

a. the alveoli become nonfunctional and cannot exchange gases
b. a chronic and irreversible blockage of the respiratory system
c. prolonged inflammation in the bronchi
d. a surgical opening in the trachea
e. insufficient oxygen in the blood
f. inflammation of the lungs
g. an infection in the nose, sinuses, and throat

DIAGRAM

137. Below is a diagram of the urinary system. Label the structures from the list under the diagram.

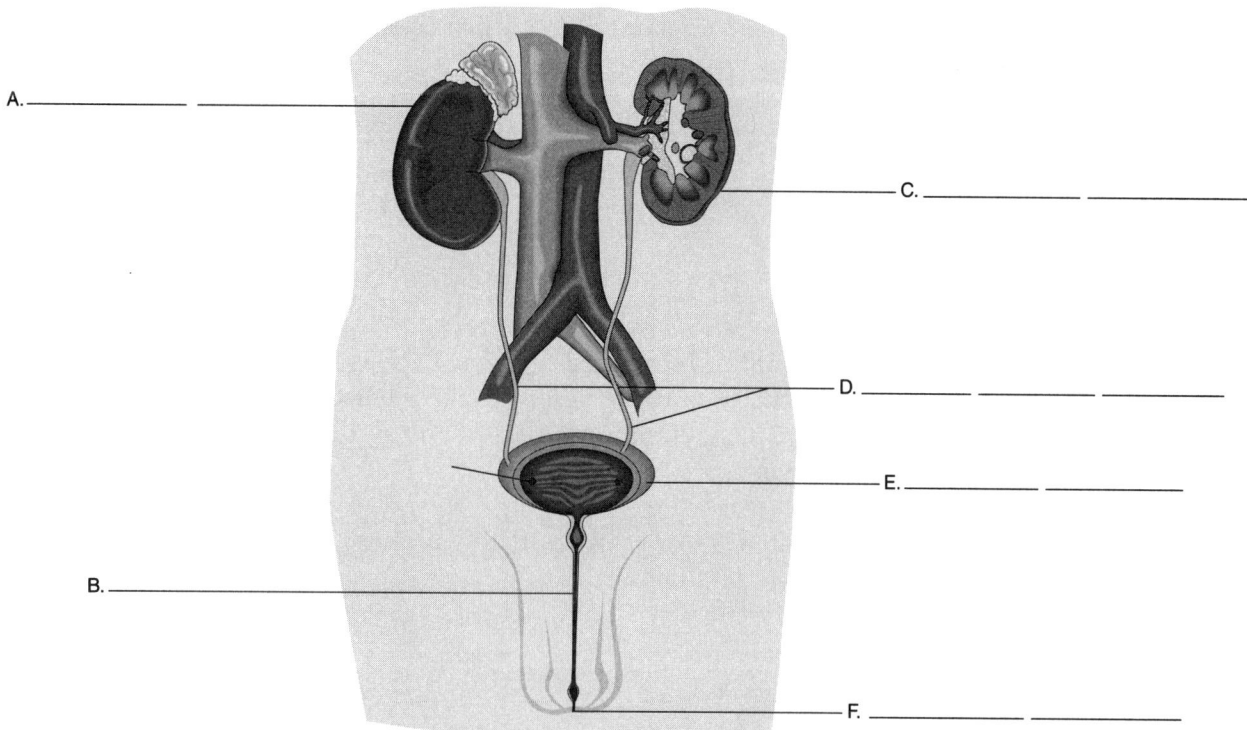

A. _____

B. _____

C. _____

D. _____

E. _____

F. _____

Figure 12-8 Diagram of the urinary system (Delmar/Cengage Learning)

right kidney   left kidney   right and left ureters
urinary bladder   urethra   urethral meatus

COMPLETION

Complete the following statements by filling in the blanks.

138. The main organs of the urinary system are the _____.

139. The kidneys remove _____ and _____ from the blood and flush them out of the body in _____.

140. After urine is produced, it travels through the _____, one from each kidney, and into the _____.

141. The brain gets a signal from the _____ to release urine once it is partially filled with _____ mL to _____ mL of urine.

142. When the bladder signals the brain to release urine, the urine travels through the _____ and out the body through the _____.

143. In males, the _____ gland sits between the bladder and the urethra.

MATCHING

Draw lines to connect each term on the left with its definition in the right column.

144. cystitis
145. nephritis
146. renal calculi
147. hydronephrosis
148. urinary incontinence

a. a buildup of fluid in the kidney because of a blocked ureter or distended bladder, which causes damage to kidney cells
b. the involuntary release of urine
c. an inflammation of the urinary bladder
d. an inflammation of the kidney
e. kidney stones

SUMMARY

Our bodies are made up of many complex, integrated systems. Each system has its own set of structures that work together. The body uses all of these structures together in order to continue its own daily functioning. Damage to any system or to part of any system will affect the body's ability to work in an efficient manner.

Chapter 13
Vitamins, Minerals, and Herbs

Learning Objectives

After completing the exercises in this chapter, you should be able to:

1. Spell and define terms.
2. Discuss the role of good nutrition in an individual's general health.
3. Give five examples of when an individual may need additional dietary supplements.
4. Describe antioxidants and phytochemicals.
5. Discuss the role of vitamin and mineral supplements in an individual's daily diet.
6. List two guidelines for the administration of herbal medications.

INTRODUCTION

The exercises you complete in this chapter will address the following key concepts from the textbook chapter:

- nutritional needs to ensure an individual's good health
- the possible need for dietary supplements
- various types of vitamin, mineral, antioxidant, and phytochemical supplements

VOCABULARY

Define the following terms.

1. obesity _____
2. vitamins _____
3. minerals _____
4. avitaminosis _____
5. hypervitaminosis _____
6. hypovitaminosis _____
7. homeostasis _____

MATCHING

Draw lines from each term on the left to its description in the right column.

8. antioxidants
9. free radicals
10. phytochemicals
11. fat-soluble vitamins
12. water-soluble vitamins
13. electrolytes

a. any one of a hundred natural chemical substances found in plants

b. acid, base, and salt particles formed by the breakdown of mineral compounds in body fluids

c. vitamins that are not stored in the body and that need to be replenished daily

d. chemical substances that neutralize free radicals

e. unstable and highly reactive molecules that can cause significant cell damage

f. vitamins that are stored in fat tissue and in the liver

LISTS

Read the following statements. Using what you have learned from the textbook, complete each list.

14. In the food we eat and the liquids we drink, there are vital nutrients that our bodies need to function. List the seven nutrients.

   a. _____
   b. _____
   c. _____
   d. _____
   e. _____

f. _____
g. _____

15. Our bodies use these nutrients in many different ways. List four ways that our bodies use nutrients.

   a. _____
   b. _____
   c. _____
   d. _____

16. Obesity is on the rise in the United States. List five health problems related to obesity.

   a. _____
   b. _____
   c. _____
   d. _____
   e. _____

17. There may be times in an individual's life when nutritional supplements are needed to keep the individual healthy and well. List five times or circumstances when an individual would need nutritional supplements.

   a. _____
   b. _____
   c. _____
   d. _____
   e. _____

COMPLETION

Complete the following statements by filling in the blanks.

18. An individual may be given a _____ for a vitamin and/or mineral supplement by her licensed health care provider. Vitamins may also be purchased as an _____ medication.

19. Just like any other prescription medication, vitamin and mineral supplements should be _____ and _____.

20. Vitamins are formed by an _____ and may come from _____ and _____ sources like vegetables, fruits, milk, and meats or from sunshine, as in vitamin D.

21. Minerals are not made by an organism. Instead they are found in _____ as well as in _____.

22. List four ways that minerals help to keep the body well and healthy.

   a. _____
   b. _____
   c. _____
   d. _____

23. Electrolytes support _____ and are vital to normal _____.

24. Antioxidants are substances that cancel the effect of free radicals. Free radicals are formed in the body as a product of _____. Free radicals are also found in the environment from substances such as _____, _____, and _____.

25. Phytochemicals may help to prevent _____ and may help to reduce damage caused by _____ such as pollution and cigarette smoke.

26. Using what you have learned from the textbook, complete the following table.

VITAMIN OR MINERAL	FUNCTION	INDICATIONS OF DEFICIENCY	TOXICITY
Vitamin A			
Vitamin D			
Vitamin E			
Vitamin C			
folic acid			
sodium			
potassium			

COMPLETION

Complete the following statements by filling in the blanks.

27. Because the use of dietary supplements has gained popularity in our society, the U.S. Congress passed the Dietary Supplement Health and Education Act (DSHEA) in 1994. List five requirements of the DSHEA.

   a. _____
   b. _____
   c. _____
   d. _____
   e. _____

28. In 2000, the FDA published a report entitled _____. This guide provides _____ _____ and _____ on dietary supplements.

29. Herbal medications and other dietary supplements are easily purchased in many different places. List four places where herbal medications and other dietary supplements may be purchased.

   a. _____
   b. _____
   c. _____
   d. _____

30. List three important facts UAPs must remember when administering herbal medications to an individual in her care.

   a. _____
   b. _____
   c. _____

Because of this, the UAP needs to report an individual's use of herbal medications to her licensed health care provider.

31. To administer herbal medications, it is recommended that the UAP have _____ _____. In some states, a licensed health care provider's order is _____ for administration. The container of herbal medication may need to be _____ by the pharmacist or licensed health care provider who is dispensing the medication.

32. Because the UAP should never administer a medication that she is unfamiliar with, the UAP needs to find a reference on herbal medications that is best for her. The most important thing to remember is that whatever reference she uses, the reference must always be _____. It must also be _____ and _____ understood.

33. List two references on herbal medications which the UAP may choose to use.

   a. _____
   b. _____

SUMMARY

Good nutrition is a key to keeping an individual healthy and well. There are times when good nutrition is not enough to keep the body healthy. Nutritional supplements may be used to provide the additional nutrients an individual needs in her diet. Understanding the benefits and risks of dietary supplements will help the UAP in her daily care of individuals and in her communication with nursing staff and licensed health care providers.

Chapter 14
Topical Medications

Learning Objectives

After completing the exercises in this chapter, you should be able to:

1. Spell and define key terms.
2. List the seven main categories of topical medications.
3. Identify the action of each main category.
4. Explain the factors that affect the absorption of topical medication.
5. Compare and contrast scabicides and pediculicides.
6. Explain the importance of paying attention to detail when applying topical medication.

INTRODUCTION

The exercises you complete in this chapter will address the following key concepts from the textbook chapter:

- the seven main categories of skin medications and what each type of medication does
- factors that affect the absorption of skin medication
- discussion of scabicides and pediculicides and what each medication is used for
- observing changes, or no changes, in skin disorders and what the UAP should do regarding these observations

VOCABULARY

Define the following terms.

1. malaise _____
2. mucous membranes _____
3. hyperglycemia _____
4. glycosuria _____
5. Cushing's syndrome _____
6. photosensitivity _____
7. herpes simplex _____
8. herpes zoster _____
9. varicella zoster _____

COMPLETION

Complete the following statements by filling in the blanks.

10. The skin is the _____ organ of the body.

11. Conditions of the skin may cause _____, _____, and general _____.

12. The treatment of choice for most skin conditions involves the use of topical medications. This involves applying medications to a _____, _____ area of the body.

13. Several factors affect how fast a topical medication will be absorbed into the body. List three factors that affect how fast a topical medication will be absorbed.

    a. _____
    b. _____
    c. _____

14. If the skin is _____, absorption of topical medications will be slower. If the skin is _____, _____ or _____ and _____, absorption will be faster.

15. To increase the absorption, the licensed health care provider might order _____ to be placed over _____ after it has been applied on the individual.

16. When the absorption needs to be slowed, the skin may be _____ to slow the absorption of the medication.

MATCHING

There are seven main classes of topical medications. Each one treats a different type of skin condition or treats a skin condition differently than another medication. Draw a line to connect each type of medication on the left with its description in the right column.

17. acne medications
18. emollients and demulcents
19. keratolytics
20. scabicides
21. pediculicides
22. antifungals
23. anti-infectives
24. antipruritics

a. used to control conditions caused by fungi
b. used to treat scabies or lice
c. used to prevent and treat infections
d. used to relieve itching
e. used to soothe irritation
f. used to control conditions of abnormal scaling or peeling of the skin
g. used to treat scabies
h. used to treat a condition of the skin most common in adolescence and early adulthood

QUESTIONS

Using what you have learned from the textbook, answer each question with one or two phrases or short sentences.

25. What are antipruritics used for?

   _____

26. What are two conditions that would be treated by antipruritics?
   a. _____
   b. _____

27. When treating skin conditions, what are corticosteroids used for?

   _____
   _____

28. What are two conditions that would be treated with corticosteroids?
   a. _____
   b. _____

29. What are emollients and demulcents used for? _____
   _____

Chapter 14 Topical Medications

30. What are two conditions that would be treated with emollients and demulcents?
    a. _____
    b. _____

31. What are keratolytics used for? _____
    _____

32. What are three conditions that would be treated with keratolytics?
    a. _____
    b. _____
    c. _____

33. What is the difference between scabies and pediculosis?
    _____
    _____

34. How are these two conditions spread? _____
    _____
    _____

35. How would it be possible to stop the indirect spread of scabies or pediculosis?
    _____
    _____

36. There are three significant adverse effects that come from frequent overuse of scabicides and pediculicides, with oral intake of these medications, or with inhalation of the vapors from these medications. What are the three significant adverse effects?
    a. _____
    b. _____
    c. _____

37. What are antifungal medications used for? _____
    _____

38. What are three conditions that would be treated with antifungals?
    a. _____
    b. _____
    c. _____

39. Good hygiene practices are very important to the healing process when treating fungal skin conditions. What are three examples of good hygiene practices?
    a. _____
    b. _____
    c. _____

40. What should the UAP do to educate an individual who is being treated for vaginitis or jock itch? _____

41. What should the UAP do to educate an individual who is being treated for athlete's foot?

42. What are the three types of anti-infective medications used to treat skin conditions?
    a.
    b.
    c.

43. What is the difference between the viruses herpes simplex and herpes zoster?

44. When treating viral conditions of the skin, topical treatment is less effective than oral treatment. However, what does topical ointment do for a viral condition of the skin?

45. Explain the difference between antiseptics and disinfectants. Give an example of each.

46. What is important for the UAP to remember when applying a burn medication?

47. List three forms of prescription and OTC antibacterial medications.
    a.
    b.
    c.

48. Acne is a condition of the skin most common in _____ and _____. Acne is usually seen on the _____, _____, _____, _____, and _____.

49. There are four grades of acne depending on its severity. _____ is the least severe. _____ is the most severe.

50. Two commonly used medications for the treatment of acne are _____ and _____.

51. In general, when using topical medications to treat skin conditions, the UAP must observe whether there is any change in the area of skin being treated. What must the UAP look for? Why? _____
_____
_____

52. Why is it important that the UAP pays attention to detail when applying topical medications? _____
_____
_____

SUMMARY

Topical medications are used to treat many different skin conditions, from mild conditions such as itching or a rash to major conditions such as skin wounds or burns. A basic understanding of skin conditions and the medications used to treat them will help the UAP to administer these medications safely and effectively to individuals who suffer from skin conditions.

Chapter 15
Eye and Ear Medications

Learning Objectives

After completing the exercises in this chapter, you should be able to:

1. Spell and define terms.
2. Discuss the uses, adverse reactions, and special considerations for various medications used to treat disorders of the eye.
3. Discuss the uses, adverse reactions, and special considerations for various medications used to treat disorders of the ear.

INTRODUCTION

The exercises you complete in this chapter will address the following key concept from the textbook chapter:

- various medications used to treat disorders of the eye
- various medications used to treat disorders of the ear

VOCABULARY

Define the following terms.

1. conjunctivitis _____
2. intraocular pressure _____
3. glaucoma _____
4. aqueous humor _____
5. myopia _____
6. otitis media _____
7. ototoxicity _____

MATCHING

There are many different types of medications used to treat disorders of the eye. Draw a line to connect each type of medication on the left with its description in the right column.

8. anti-inflammatory medications
9. antiglaucoma medications
10. anti-infectives
11. mydriatics
12. local anesthetics

a. used to dilate the pupil prior to an ophthalmic exam
b. used topically on the eye before a minor surgical procedure, before removing foreign bodies from the eye, or to decrease pain from an injury
c. used to relieve inflammation of the eye
d. used to lower intraocular pressure
e. used to treat bacterial infections in the eye

COMPLETION

Complete the following statements by filling in the blanks.

13. If there is no improvement in 2 to 3 days of beginning treatment for an eye infection, the UAP should _____.

14. Anti-inflammatory medications are used to _____ from allergic reactions, burns, or irritation from a foreign substance.

15. Eyedrops and ointments are administered into the _____ of the eye.

16. If an individual who is receiving an anti-infective medication complains of burning and/or itching in the eye, the UAP should _____
_____
_____

QUESTIONS

Using what you have learned from the textbook, answer each question with one or two phrases or short sentences.

17. When treating the eye, what are corticosteroids used for?
   _____

18. What types of medications are used to treat the eye after cataract surgery?
   _____

19. What do antiglaucoma medications do? _____
   _____

20. What effect might antiglaucoma medications have on an individual's blood pressure and pulse? _____

21. Local anesthetics are applied to the eye topically before a minor surgical procedure. What should the UAP do to protect the eye until the individual regains her blink reflex?
   _____
   _____

MATCHING

This chapter discusses six categories of medications used to treat disorders of the ear. Draw a line to connect each type of medication on the left with its description in the right column.

22. anti-inflammatory medications
23. antibacterials
24. antifungals
25. local analgesics
26. local anesthetics
27. wax emulsifiers

a. used to remove a buildup of wax from an individual's ear(s)

b. used in combination with anesthetics to treat congestion, pain, and swelling

c. used in combination with analgesics to treat congestion, pain, and swelling

d. used to treat fungal infections and some bacterial infections of the ear

e. used to decrease redness, swelling, and pain caused by the body's reaction to infection

f. used to treat bacterial infections of the ear

SUMMARY

There are many different types of eye and ear medications available to treat various disorders of the eye and ear. A basic understanding of these disorders and medications will help the UAP to administer eye and ear medications more safely and effectively to individuals who suffer from eye and ear disorders.

Chapter 16
Psychotropic Medications

Learning Objectives

After completing the exercises in this chapter, you should be able to:

1. Spell and define terms.
2. Describe the five classes of psychotropic medications.
3. Discuss the uses, adverse reactions, and special considerations for selected psychotropic medications.
4. Describe extrapyramidal symptoms, pseudoparkinsonism, and tardive dyskinesia.

INTRODUCTION

The exercises you complete in this chapter will address the following key concepts from the textbook chapter:

- the five main classes of psychotropic medications
- administration of various psychotropic medications
- symptoms of adverse reactions to various psychotropic medications

VOCABULARY

Define the following terms.

1. mental health _____
2. psychotropic medications _____
3. psychotic behavior _____
4. ataxia _____
5. diaphoresis _____
6. paralytic ileus _____
7. agoraphobia _____
8. hysteroid dysphoria _____
9. dysuria _____
10. polyuria _____
11. nystagmus _____
12. extrapyramidal symptoms _____
13. pseudoparkinsonism _____
14. tardive dyskinesia _____

COMPLETION

Complete the following statements by filling in the blanks.

15. An individual's mental health may affect his _____ and _____ well-being.

16. List four possible causes of mental illness.
    a. _____
    b. _____
    c. _____
    d. _____

17. Psychotropic medications do not cure mental illness. They help to _____ of mental or emotional illness in an individual's life.

18. Psychotropic medications are usually used in combination with other treatments, including _____ or _____.

19. There are five classes of psychotropic medications. List the five classes of these medications. Give a brief explanation of what each one does.

    a. _____

    b. _____

    c. _____

    d. _____

    e. _____

20. Central nervous system (CNS) stimulants are medications that improve the function of the central nervous system. These medications are used to treat _____, _____, and _____.

21. _____ and _____ are two types of central nervous system (CNS) stimulants.

22. Anxiety is a _____.

23. There are many different signs of anxiety. List four of the signs of anxiety.

    a. _____
    b. _____
    c. _____
    d. _____

24. Medications commonly used to treat anxiety are called _____.

QUESTIONS

Using what you have learned from the textbook, answer each question with one or two phrases or short sentences.

25. How do individuals demonstrate the symptoms of depression?

26. Is depression a normal occurrence as an individual goes through life? How should it be treated? _____

27. What are four of the symptoms of clinical depression?

    a. _____
    b. _____
    c. _____
    d. _____

28. About how long does it take for antidepressant medications to have a noticeable effect on an individual? _____

COMPLETION

Complete the following statements by filling in the blanks.

29. Lithium is the primary medication used to treat the _____ phase of _____.

30. Bipolar disorder was previously called _____ or _____.

31. Lithium intoxication may occur if lithium levels are too high in the body. There are many early signs of lithium intoxication. List eight of the early signs.
    a. _____
    b. _____
    c. _____
    d. _____
    e. _____
    f. _____
    g. _____
    h. _____

32. List the four signs that indicate an advanced case of lithium toxicity.
    a. _____
    b. _____
    c. _____
    d. _____

33. If the UAP notices any of these symptoms in an individual taking lithium, he should _____.

34. Antipsychotic medications, or neuroleptics, are used to modify _____.

35. List the four types of mental illness that neuroleptics are used to treat.
    a. _____
    b. _____
    c. _____
    d. _____

MATCHING

There are many physical adverse reactions to neuroleptics. Draw lines to connect each physical symptom on the left to its description in the right column.

36. torticollis
37. carpopedal spasms
38. trismus
39. oculogyric crisis
40. protrusion

a. a decrease in spontaneous movement
b. spasms and rigidity in various muscle groups
c. involuntary movements of the face, trunk, and extremities that develop as a side effect of long-term neuroleptic use

41. akathisia

42. dystonia

43. bradykinesia

44. tardive dyskinesia

d. a muscle spasm of the neck in which the head is pulled to one side and turned so that the chin is pointing to the other side of the body

e. spasms and rigidity in the hands and feet

f. severe and repeated upward rolling of the eyeballs

g. sticking out of the tongue

h. spasms in the jaw muscles

i. an inability to sit down; agitation, fidgeting, pacing

SUMMARY

Psychotropic medications are a complex group of medications with a number of unusual side effects. The UAP needs to be observant for any and all changes in an individual. The UAP needs to recognize any unusual reaction and report it to the licensed health care provider in a timely fashion. Available references need to be used by the UAP to gain a basic understanding for each type of medication and used to answer any questions before a medication is given.

Chapter 17
Analgesics and Anesthetics

Learning Objectives

After completing the exercises in this chapter, you should be able to:

1. Spell and define terms.
2. Discuss the uses, adverse reactions, and special considerations for analgesics, anesthetics, hypnotics, and sedatives.
3. Lists three ways pain affects an individual's quality of life.
4. Describe a pain assessment scale.
5. List six signs of pain the UAP should look for in an individual with dementia or who is in a coma.

INTRODUCTION

The exercises you complete in this chapter will address the following key concepts from the textbook chapter:

- various medications used to relieve or prevent pain and to treat insomnia and anxiety
- types of pain and how they affect an individual's quality of life
- pain assessment scales including ways to assess for pain with individuals who have dementia or are in a coma

VOCABULARY

Define the following terms.

1. acute pain _____
2. addiction _____
3. asthenia _____
4. chronic pain _____
5. euphoria _____
6. migraines _____
7. paresthesias _____
8. somnolence _____
9. tinnitus _____
10. tolerance _____

MATCHING

There are many different medications used to relieve or prevent pain and to treat insomnia and anxiety. Draw a line to match each type of medication on the left with its description for use in the right column.

11. analgesics
12. opiates
13. analgesic-antipyretics
14. sedatives
15. hypnotics
16. antimigraine medications
17. anesthetics

a. used to cause sleep
b. used to calm, soothe, or quiet without causing sleep
c. used to relieve pain caused by many different conditions
d. used in the relief of moderate to severe pain; also called opioids
e. used to treat migraine headaches
f. used to prevent pain, relax muscles, and induce lack of sensation
g. used to relieve mild to moderate pain and reduce fever

COMPLETION

Complete the following statements by filling in the blanks.

18. The nervous system controls and coordinates all body activities. The nervous system is made up of three parts. These are:

    a. _____

    b. _____

    c. _____

19. Pain is defined as _____ .

20. Because of the effects pain has on the quality of an individual's life, it is considered the _____ .

MATCHING

There are four types of pain. Draw a line to match each type of pain on the left with its description in the right column.

21. acute pain
22. chronic pain
23. phantom pain
24. radiating pain

a. Lasts longer than six months. May be caused from multiple medical conditions.

b. Moves from place of origin to other places, for instance, chest pain moving to the arm or jaw.

c. Occurs suddenly and without warning. Usually is the result of injury or surgery. Decreases over time as healing takes place.

d. Is the result of an amputation. Pain is real, not imaginary.

COMPLETION

Complete the following statements by filling in the blanks.

25. UAPs have an important role of observing the individuals in their care for pain and for medicating the individuals as ordered. _____ _____ may be used to help the UAP to determine the amount of pain an individual is experiencing. This may be used with children, adults, and individuals who do not speak or understand English.

26. When caring for an individual who is unable to communicate the amount of pain she is experiencing, such as an individual with dementia or who is in a coma, the UAP needs to observe for signs of pain. List six signs of pain the UAP should look for.

    a. _____

    b. _____

    c. _____

    d. _____

    e. _____

    h. _____

27. The best way to control an individual's pain is by preventing pain from developing or worsening. To do this, the UAP should administer an individual's medication _____.

QUESTIONS

28. Approximately 30 to 60 minutes after medicating an individual for pain, the UAP needs to observe the individual. What is the UAP looking for?
    a. _____
    b. _____

29. If the medication is not effective or if the individual is experiencing adverse effects, what should the UAP do?
    _____.

COMPLETION

30. Analgesics are medications used to relieve pain caused by many different conditions. List the three classes of analgesics.
    a. _____
    b. _____
    c. _____

31. Opiates, also called opioids, are used in the relief of moderate to severe pain. The medication _____ or _____ works to reverse the effects of opiates.

32. List three effects of opioids on the body.
    a. _____
    b. _____
    c. _____

33. Analgesic-antipyretics are also known as nonnarcotic and nonopioid analgesics. Many analgesic-antipyretics are available over-the-counter. List three reasons why analgesic-antipyretics may be used.
    a. _____
    b. _____
    c. _____

34. Individuals on long-term salicylate treatment need to be monitored for side effects, especially older adults who are at risk for _____ and _____ _____, which may be "silent."

35. Although acetaminophen has fewer side effects than salicylates, acetaminophen may cause _____ even with only a single dose and may cause _____ _____ especially if the individual is also drinking alcohol or taking other acetaminophen-containing medications.

36. _____ _____ are medications that are used to treat conditions other than pain. When combined with narcotic analgesics and analgesic-antipyretics, however, these medications increase the analgesic effect of the medications.

37. Two classes of these medications commonly used for analgesia are:

    a. _____

    b. _____

QUESTIONS

Using what you have learned from the textbook, answer each question with one or two phrases or short sentences.

38. What causes migraine headaches?

    _____

    _____

39. What are three symptoms of a migraine headache?

    a. _____

    b. _____

    c. _____

40. What are anesthetics used for?

    a. _____

    b. _____

    c. _____

41. There are three main types of anesthetics. What are they?

    a. _____

    b. _____

    c. _____

42. Sedatives and hypnotics are used to treat disorders that cause anxiety and insomnia. What is the difference between sedatives and hypnotics?

    _____

    _____

43. What is a significant concern when an individual is taking barbiturates?

    _____

44. What are two signs of respiratory dysfunction in an individual who is taking barbiturates?

    a. _____

    b. _____

45. There are seven signs of toxicity that may occur when an individual is taking barbiturates. List four of those signs.

a. _____

b. _____

c. _____

d. _____

46. What should the UAP do if she observes either respiratory dysfunction or toxicity in an individual who is taking barbiturates? _____

_____

_____

SUMMARY

Pain, insomnia, and anxiety can all negatively affect an individual's quality of life. The UAP can help an individual function to her highest potential and live her life to the fullest by administering these medications as ordered and reporting side effects and adverse effects immediately to an individual's licensed HCP.

Chapter 18
Antiparkinsonian Medications, Anticonvulsants, and Medications for Treating Alzheimer's Disease

Learning Objectives

After reading this chapter and completing the review questions, you should be able to:

1. Spell and define terms.
2. Discuss the uses, adverse reactions, and special considerations for various medications used to treat seizure disorders, Parkinson's disease, and Alzheimer's disease.
3. State the mood changes that occur in an individual with Alzheimer's disease.

Chapter 18 Antiparkinsonian Medications, Anticonvulsants, and Medications for Treating Alzheimer's Disease

INTRODUCTION

The exercises you complete in this chapter will address the following key concepts from the textbook chapter:

- medications used to treat seizure disorders
- medications used to treat symptoms of Parkinson's disease
- medications used to treat symptoms of Alzheimer's disease
- mood changes that may be seen in an individual who has Alzheimer's disease

VOCABULARY

Define the following terms.

1. Alzheimer's disease _____
2. vertigo _____
3. epilepsy _____
4. status epilepticus _____
5. syncope _____

COMPLETION

Complete the following statements by filling in the blanks.

6. Anticonvulsants are medications used to treat _____.

7. According to the Epilepsy Foundation, more than _____ Americans of all ages have epilepsy. Approximately _____ additional new cases of seizure disorders and epilepsy are diagnosed each year. Over their lifetime, ___ in ___ adults in the United States will have a seizure.

8. The goal of anticonvulsant therapy is _____.

9. An individual's daily dose of anticonvulsant medication is adjusted based upon _____.

QUESTIONS

Using what you have learned from the textbook, answer each question with one or two phrases or short sentences.

10. What are three adverse reactions of anticonvulsant medications?
    a. _____
    b. _____
    c. _____

11. Why should anticonvulsant medications never be suddenly stopped or omitted (skipped)?
    _____

12. What is Parkinson's disease? _____
   _____
   _____

13. What type of medication is used to treat Parkinson's disease?
   _____

COMPLETION

Complete the following statements by filling in the blanks.

14. There are approximately _____ individuals in the United States with Parkinson's disease. Two-thirds (2/3) of these individuals develop the disease between the ages of __ and __.

15. List the four symptoms of Parkinson's disease.
   a. _____
   b. _____
   c. _____
   d. _____

16. Sinemet is used most often for the long-term treatment of Parkinson's disease. Sinemet is recommended as the initial treatment for individuals _____ and individuals with _____.

17. List five adverse reactions to Sinemet.
   a. _____
   b. _____
   c. _____
   d. _____
   e. _____

QUESTIONS

Using what you have learned from the textbook, answer each question with one or two phrases or short sentences.

18. Why are dopamine agonists used along with levodopa (Sinemet)?
   _____

19. Why do antiparkinsonian medications need to be tapered off for 1 to 2 weeks rather than being stopped quickly?
   _____

COMPLETION

Complete the following statements by filling in the blanks.

20. Alzheimer's disease is the most common form of dementia. Four million Americans are currently affected by Alzheimer's disease. It is estimated that by 2030 as many as _____ Americans will have the disease (Broyles et al., 2007).

21. Alzheimer's disease causes _____.

22. At this time the cause of Alzheimer's disease is _____.

23. List five of the behavioral problems of Alzheimer's disease.

    a. _____

    b. _____

    c. _____

    d. _____

    e. _____

QUESTIONS

Using what you have learned from the textbook, answer each question with one or two phrases or short sentences.

24. What are the two classes of medications that are being used today for the treatment of Alzheimer's disease?

    a. _____

    b. _____

25. Which medication used for the treatment of Alzheimer's disease can cause significant liver toxicity? _____

26. Which medication has been approved for the treatment of moderate to severe Alzheimer's disease? _____

SUMMARY

A seizure disorder, Parkinson's disease, or Alzheimer's disease all have a significant impact on an individual's life. Medications to control seizures or symptoms of these diseases play a role in determining the quality of the individual's life. A basic understanding of these illnesses and the medications used to treat them will help the UAP to administer medications safely and effectively to those who suffer from these disorders and will help to ensure that the individual has the best quality of life possible.

Chapter 19
Medications for Treating Infections

Learning Objectives

After completing the exercises in this chapter, you should be able to:

1. Spell and define terms.
2. Describe how infection occurs.
3. Name at least three infectious diseases.
4. List the signs of a serious infection.
5. List the emergency supplies and medications that should be available when administering medication to an individual.
6. Describe various types of antimicrobials used to treat infection along with adverse reactions and special considerations for these medications.
7. Describe the various types of antifungal medications along with adverse reactions and special considerations for these medications.
8. Describe the various types of antiviral and antiretroviral medications along with adverse reactions and special considerations for these medications.
9. Discuss the symptoms and treatment of tuberculosis.
10. State the general recommendations for immunization.

INTRODUCTION

The exercises you complete in this chapter will address the following key concepts from the textbook chapter:

- how an infection occurs
- the danger signs of a serious infection
- emergency supplies and medications for the treatment of an allergic reaction or anaphylactic shock
- various types of medications used to treat infections
- examples of common viruses and fungal diseases
- various types of medications used to treat viruses, fungal infections, and HIV/AIDS
- symptoms and treatment of tuberculosis
- recommendations for immunization

VOCABULARY

Define the following terms.

1. microorganism _____
2. drug-resistant organism _____
3. antibiotics _____
4. culture _____
5. allergic reaction _____
6. anaphylactic shock _____
7. virus _____
8. fungus _____
9. tinnitus _____
10. orthostatic hypotension _____
11. local anesthesia _____
12. hypesthesia _____
13. HIV _____
14. pancreatitis _____
15. immunity _____
16. immunization _____

COMPLETION

Complete the following statements by filling in the blanks.

17. Infectious diseases may be caused by _____, _____, _____, _____, or other microorganisms.

18. An infection happens when microorganisms _____ the body or a body part, _____, and produce _____ or _____.

19. There has been an increase in drug-resistant microorganisms in recent years. Researchers say that this is partly due to _____ of antibiotics.

20. Give two examples of organisms resistant to most antimicrobials.
    a. _____
    b. _____

21. List seven warning signs of a serious infection.
    a. _____
    b. _____
    c. _____
    d. _____
    e. _____
    f. _____
    g. _____

22. List eight ways the UAP may minimize her risk of developing an infection.
    a. _____
    b. _____
    c. _____
    d. _____
    e. _____
    f. _____
    g. _____
    h. _____

23. Medication may cause a _____ even if the individual taking the medication does not have any known allergies.

24. After giving an antibiotic, the UAP must always _____ the individual for at least _____ minutes to check for any unusual reaction.

25. There are seven different emergency supplies that the UAP should have readily available whenever she gives a medication. These emergency supplies may be needed if an individual goes into anaphylactic shock. List the seven emergency supplies.
    a. _____
    b. _____
    c. _____
    d. _____
    e. _____
    f. _____
    g. _____

26. List the six major groups of antibiotics.
    a. _____
    b. _____
    c. _____
    d. _____
    e. _____
    f. _____

27. Antibiotics are a type of medication used to treat infectious diseases. List six diseases that are treated with antibiotics.
    a. _____
    b. _____
    c. _____
    d. _____
    e. _____
    f. _____

28. Aminoglycosides may cause toxicity. List six signs of aminoglycoside toxicity.
    a. _____
    b. _____
    c. _____
    d. _____
    e. _____
    f. _____

29. The most common adverse reaction to penicillin is _____.

30. Zyvox is a new class of antibiotics. It is used mainly in an institutional setting. Zyvox kills bacteria by stopping protein development. What group of antibiotics does it belong to?
    _____

31. A fungus is a plantlike organism such as a mold or yeast. List three common fungal diseases.
    a. _____
    b. _____
    c. _____

32. Antifungal medications work by killing fungal cells. Antifungal medications do not work against _____, _____, or _____.

QUESTIONS

Using what you have learned from the textbook, answer each question with one or two phrases or short sentences.

33. What should the UAP tell an individual who is being treated for a vaginal fungal infection? _____

34. When educating an individual who is being treated for a vaginal fungal infection caused by Candida, what specifically should the UAP instruct her on?

    a. _____
    b. _____
    c. _____
    d. _____

35. What is a virus? _____

36. What are six common viruses?

    a. _____
    b. _____
    c. _____
    d. _____
    e. _____
    f. _____

37. Acyclovir is an antiviral agent used to treat genital herpes. How does it affect outbreaks of genital herpes? _____

38. What should the UAP tell an individual who is being treated for genital herpes about sexual intercourse? _____

39. Famciclovir is used to treat two types of herpes. What are the two types?

    a. _____
    b. _____

40. What two antiviral agents work against influenza A?

    a. _____
    b. _____

41. What are two other uses for amantadine hydrochloride?

    a. _____
    b. _____

42. Antiretroviral medications are used to treat HIV, the virus that causes AIDS. What is important to remember about the adverse effects of antiretroviral medications? _____

43. What is tuberculosis (TB)? _____

44. How is tuberculosis spread? _____

_____

45. What are the symptoms of tuberculosis?

a. _____
b. _____
c. _____
d. _____
e. _____
f. _____
g. _____

46. How is tuberculosis treated and for how long?

_____

_____

COMPLETION

Complete the following statements by filling in the blanks.

47. Define the term *helminthiasis*. _____

48. List the four types of parasitic worms that infest humans.

a. _____
b. _____
c. _____
d. _____

49. List four instructions to give the individual being treated for parasitic worms to avoid reinfestation.

a. _____
b. _____
c. _____
d. _____

50. List five diseases caused by protozoa.

a. _____
b. _____
c. _____
d. _____
e. _____

51. Define the term *opportunistic*. _____

52. What information should the UAP emphasize when educating an individual who is taking an antiprotozoal agent? _____

53. Immunity is built up in the body through a mechanism called the _____.

54. An organism of some type called an _____ enters the body and triggers a series of complex activities.

55. Mechanical and chemical forces form _____ in plasma cells to fight the _____ and prevent further illness.

56. List the four things that immunity does for the body.

   a. _____
   b. _____
   c. _____
   d. _____

57. Active immunization occurs when a _____ or _____ is given, causing the body to form _____.

58. Passive immunization occurs when a _____ _____ or _____ is given so that the body does not have to produce it.

59. Briefly explain the benefits and risks of getting a vaccine or immunization.

   _____
   _____

SUMMARY

Infectious diseases are the number one killer of human beings in the world. The UAP needs to know how to avoid getting an infection or passing on an infection to another individual. It is also important for the UAP to understand the causes and treatments of various infections so that the UAP can give the most effective care possible to the individuals with whom she works.

Chapter 20
Medications for Treating Cancer

Learning Objectives

After completing the exercises in this chapter, you should be able to:

1. Spell and define terms.
2. Discuss the uses of chemotherapy in treating cancer, along with side effects and adverse reactions.
3. Explain the care of individuals being treated for cancer.
4. Define other methods of treatment for an individual who has cancer.

INTRODUCTION

The exercises you complete in this chapter will address the following key concepts from the textbook chapter:

- chemotherapy and its effects on the human body
- techniques that the UAP should use when caring for an individual who has cancer
- other methods of treatment for an individual who has cancer

VOCABULARY

Define the following terms.

1. malignant cells _____
2. metastasis _____
3. chemotherapy _____
4. remission _____
5. exacerbation _____
6. antiangiogenesis _____
7. brachytherapy _____
8. gene therapy _____
9. hyperthermia _____
10. petechiae _____
11. immunotherapy _____
12. thermal ablation _____
13. targeted therapy _____
14. photodynamic therapy (PDT) _____
15. anorexia _____

COMPLETION

Complete the following statements by filling in the blanks.

16. According to the American Cancer Society, cancer of some type affects ____ out of ____ men and ____ out of ____ women in the United States.

17. The key to the successful treatment of cancer is _____ (American Cancer Society, 2009b).

18. Cancer spreads quickly in the human body because of a mechanism called _____.

19. When malignant cells metastasize, they _____ and _____ normal cells.

20. Today individuals with cancer have numerous options for treatment. List four options available to an individual.
    a. _____
    b. _____
    c. _____
    d. _____

21. The type of treatment administered to an individual by his licensed HCP depends upon five factors. List the five factors.
    a. _____
    b. _____
    c. _____
    d. _____
    e. _____

22. Chemotherapy uses medications that destroy cells. List two instances in cancer treatment where chemotherapy would be used.
    a. _____
    b. _____

QUESTIONS

Using what you have learned in the textbook, answer each question with one or two phrases or short sentences.

23. The medications used in chemotherapy are called antineoplastic medications. The medications work by killing malignant cells. What other types of normal cells do they kill? _____

24. What is the goal of chemotherapy? _____

25. Explain the term *remission*. _____

26. What is the main difficulty with antineoplastic medications? _____

COMPLETION

Complete the following statements by filling in the blanks.

27. When an individual is receiving chemotherapy treatment, it is important to keep the environment as free from potentially infectious microorganisms as possible. List four ways the UAP may maintain the cleanest environment possible.
    a. _____
    b. _____
    c. _____
    d. _____

168 Module 4 Medications and Their Effects on the Body

28. Chemotherapy treatment may cause anorexia, nausea and vomiting, and inflammation of the mouth and mucous membranes. List five ways in which the UAP may provide for an individual's nutritional needs when that individual is receiving chemotherapy treatments.

    a. _____
    b. _____
    c. _____
    d. _____
    e. _____

29. List three other ways in which the UAP may give care to an individual who is receiving chemotherapy treatments.

    a. _____
    b. _____
    c. _____

QUESTIONS

Using what you have learned from the textbook, answer each question with one or two phrases or short sentences.

30. What are petechiae a sign of? _____

31. Nausea and vomiting are common adverse reactions to chemotherapy. What type of medications may control these symptoms? _____

32. What is the goal of radiation therapy? _____

33. How is radiation therapy administered?

    a. _____
    b. _____
    c. _____

34. What are the benefits of radiation therapy over chemotherapy? _____

35. What is the main goal of surgery in treating cancer? _____

36. What is another use for surgery in treating cancer? _____

37. How does immunotherapy work in treating cancer? _____

38. Describe the two main ways in which hyperthermia may be used.

    a. _____
    b. _____

39. How does antiangiogenesis work? _____
_____

SUMMARY

Cancer and its treatments may affect an individual physically, mentally, and emotionally, causing him to be very tired and weak. By understanding the mechanism of cancer and cancer treatments, the UAP may provide the care needed to help the individual at every level of his daily life.

Chapter 21
Medications for Treating Cardiovascular Disorders

Learning Objectives

After completing the exercises in this chapter, you should be able to:

1. Spell and define terms.
2. List the warning signs of a heart attack.
3. State two primary causes of chest pain.
4. State the uses, adverse reactions, and special considerations of various medications used to treat cardiovascular disorders.

INTRODUCTION

The exercises you complete in this chapter will address the following key concepts from the textbook chapter:

- warning signs of a heart attack
- primary causes of chest pain
- various medications used to treat and manage cardiovascular disorders

VOCABULARY

Define the following terms.

1. angina pectoris _____
2. myocardial infarction _____
3. arrhythmia _____
4. angioedema _____
5. thrombus _____
6. embolus _____
7. arteriosclerosis _____
8. cardiomyopathy _____
9. myalgia _____
10. myopathy _____

COMPLETION

Complete the following statements by filling in the blanks.

11. Coronary heart disease is currently the _____ cause of death in the United States.

12. Chest pain may be caused by a number of different factors. List three factors that may cause chest pain.

    a. _____
    b. _____
    c. _____

13. There are many different risk factors for chest pain and possible heart attack. List five of the risk factors for chest pain and possible heart attack.

    a. _____
    b. _____
    c. _____
    d. _____
    e. _____

14. List three symptoms of a heart attack.
    a. _____
    b. _____
    c. _____
15. If a UAP notices that an individual is having symptoms of a heart attack, she should call _____ or the _____ immediately.
16. Many individuals die from a heart attack because they _____.
17. Cardiovascular medications are used to treat disorders that affect the _____, _____ _____, and _____.

QUESTIONS

Using what you have learned from the textbook, answer each question with one or two phrases or short sentences.

18. What do Cardiac glycosides do?
    a. _____
    b. _____
    c. _____
19. What is the most commonly used cardiac glycoside? _____
20. Digitalis toxicity is a type of adverse reaction to digitalis preparations. What are the most common early symptoms of digitalis toxicity?
    a. _____
    b. _____
    c. _____
    d. _____

MATCHING

There are many different types of cardiovascular medications. Draw a line from the medication type on the left to its description of how it works in the right column.

21. cardiac glycosides
22. antiarrhythmics
23. vasodilators
24. vasoconstrictors
25. antihypertensives
26. antilipidemic
27. anticoagulants
28. platelet inhibitors
29. thrombolytics

a. treat high blood pressure
b. stop platelets from sticking together to form clots
c. treat iron-deficiency anemia and megaloblastic anemia
d. lower high blood levels of fatty substances
e. stimulate bone marrow to make more red blood cells
f. dilate blood vessels and increase blood flow
g. used to treat an irregular heart beat

30. colony-stimulating factors (CSFS)
31. medications to treat anemia

h. strengthen and improve the contractions of the heart muscle, slow the heart beat
i. dissolve clots
j. constrict blood vessels and increase blood pressure
k. prevent or delay clotting of the blood

QUESTIONS

Using what you have learned from the textbook, answer each question with one or two phrases or short sentences.

32. What are the risks of leaving high blood pressure untreated? _____

33. Certain medications should not be administered with grapefruit juice. What are two cardiovascular medications that should *not* be administered with grapefruit juice?
    a. _____
    b. _____

34. What are the risks of having high blood levels of lipids (fatty substances)?
    a. _____
    b. _____
    c. _____
    d. _____

35. What is the difference between a thrombus and an embolus?
    _____
    _____

36. Do anticoagulants dissolve blood clots? ❏ Yes ❏ No If yes, how do anticoagulants dissolve clots? If no, how do anticoagulants work?
    _____
    _____

37. When are anticoagulants used?
    a. _____
    b. _____
    c. _____

38. What is "purple-toe" syndrome? _____
    _____

39. Because certain cardiovascular medications are administered by injection, these medications may only be administered by licensed health care providers. What are three cardiovascular medications that must be administered only by licensed HCPs?
    a. _____
    b. _____
    c. _____

SUMMARY

The cardiovascular system is one of the vital systems in the body. Keeping this body system healthy will help to keep an individual healthy. It is the UAP's responsibility to have a basic knowledge of medications used to keep the cardiovascular system healthy. In addition, the UAP must be able to observe and report any unusual circumstances that may arise while she is giving care.

Chapter 22
Medications for Treating Endocrine Disorders

Learning Objectives

After completing the exercises in this chapter, you should be able to:
1. Spell and define terms.
2. Discuss the uses, adverse reactions, and special considerations for various medications used to treat endocrine system disorders.
3. Describe diabetes mellitus and give the warning signs.
4. State signs and symptoms of hypoglycemia and hyperglycemia.

INTRODUCTION

The exercises you complete in this chapter will address the following key concepts from the textbook chapter:

- various medications used to treat endocrine system disorders
- warning signs of diabetes mellitus
- warning signs and symptoms of hypoglycemia and hyperglycemia

VOCABULARY

Define the following terms.

1. hormone _____
2. diabetes mellitus _____
3. hypoglycemia _____
4. hyperglycemia _____
5. lactic acidosis _____
6. thrombophlebitis _____

COMPLETION

Complete the following statements by filling in the blanks.

7. The endocrine system contains glands that produce hormones to control _____ and regulate _____ _____. If these glands make too much or too little of the hormones they produce, _____ result.

8. The endocrine system is made up eight glands. Name five of the eight glands that make up the endocrine system.

   a. _____
   b. _____
   c. _____
   d. _____
   e. _____

9. The adrenal glands make hormones known as corticosteroids. Corticosteroids help the body to:

   a. _____
   b. _____
   c. _____
   d. _____

10. Treatment with adrenal corticosteroids is supportive, not _____.

11. Name two adrenal corticosteroids. _____

12. The islets of Langerhans in the pancreas produce insulin. The three major conditions related to insulin are _____, _____, and _____.

13. Oral antidiabetic medications are used to manage and treat _____ _____, also known as _____.

QUESTIONS

Using what you have learned from the textbook, answer each question with one or two phrases or short sentences.

14. How are oral antidiabetic medications administered?
    _____
    _____

15. When are oral antidiabetic medications administered?
    _____
    _____

16. There are a number of warning signs and symptoms of diabetes mellitus. What are five of the warning signs and symptoms of diabetes mellitus?
    a. _____
    b. _____
    c. _____
    d. _____
    e. _____

17. There are a number of warning signs and symptoms of hypoglycemia. What are five of the warning signs and symptoms of hypoglycemia?
    a. _____
    b. _____
    c. _____
    d. _____
    e. _____

18. There are a number of warning signs and symptoms of hyperglycemia. What are five of the warning signs and symptoms of hyperglycemia?
    a. _____
    b. _____
    c. _____
    d. _____
    e. _____

Remember, if the UAP observes signs or symptoms of hypoglycemia or hyperglycemia in an individual for whom she is caring, she must report them to the individual's licensed health care provider right away.

MATCHING

Oral antidiabetic medications are used to manage and treat non-insulin-dependent diabetes mellitus (NIDDM), Type 2 diabetes. Draw a line to connect the oral antidiabetic medication on the left with its related information on the right.

19. sulfonylureas

20. biguanides

21. thiazolidinediones

22. alpha glucosidase inhibitors (Precose)

23. meglitinides

24. Proglycem

a. take with the first bite of food at each meal.

b. used to treat severe hypoglycemia

c. stimulate the cells in the pancreas to make insulin

d. use alone or with sulfonylureas, metformin, or insulin

e. may cause lactic acidosis

f. used to increase insulin production from the cells of the pancreas and improve insulin activity in the body

QUESTIONS

Using what you have learned from the textbook, answer each question with one or two phrases or short sentences.

25. What are thyroid hormones used for?

    a. _____
    b. _____

26. Treatment with thyroid hormones needs to continue for the life of the individual. Lab work should be done periodically by the individual's licensed HCP. Why does lab work need to be routinely done?

    a. _____
    b. _____

27. Adverse reactions of thyroid medication are usually due to an overdose resulting in toxicity. What are eight signs and symptoms of toxicity?

    a. _____
    b. _____
    c. _____
    d. _____
    e. _____
    f. _____
    g. _____
    h. _____

28. What are antithyroid hormones used for?
    a. _____
    b. _____
29. Why is the liquid iodine preparation diluted (mixed) with water or juice and then administered through a straw? _____

SUMMARY

Endocrine system disorders may range from growth disorders to issues with unstable blood sugars, including diabetes mellitus. A basic understanding of these illnesses and the medications used to treat them will help the UAP to administer medications safely and effectively to individuals with disorders of the endocrine system.

Chapter 23
Medications for Treating Gastrointestinal Disorders

Learning Objectives

After completing the exercises in this chapter, you should be able to:

1. Spell and define terms.
2. Identify causes of gastrointestinal disorders.
3. Discuss the uses, adverse reactions, and special considerations for various gastrointestinal medications.

Chapter 23 Medications for Treating Gastrointestinal Disorders

INTRODUCTION

The exercises you complete in this chapter will address the following key concepts from the textbook chapter:

- causes of various gastrointestinal disorders
- medications used to treat various gastrointestinal disorders

VOCABULARY

Define the following terms.

1. erosive esophagitis _____
2. pyrosis _____
3. ulcer _____
4. rebound hyperacidity _____
5. peristalsis _____

MATCHING

There are many different types of medications used to treat GI disorders. Each one does something different. Draw lines to connect each type of medication on the left with its description in the right column.

6. antacids
7. histamine H_2-receptor antagonists
8. GI protectants
9. proton pump
10. medications to treat *H. pylori*
11. antidiarrhea
12. antiflatulents
13. laxatives
14. antiemetics
15. emetics

a. decrease the number of loose, watery stools
b. induce vomiting in an individual who has taken an overdose of oral drugs or has ingested certain poisons
c. used to treat vomiting, vertigo, motion sickness, and nausea due to chemotherapy
d. neutralize hydrochloric acid in the stomach inhibitors
e. protect the lining of the stomach
f. decrease the secretion of gastric acid medications
g. treats *H. pylori*
h. used for short-term treatment of ulcers and other GI disorders
i. break up gas bubbles in the GI tract
j. aid the body in the elimination of waste

COMPLETION

Complete the following statements by filling in the blanks.

16. There are many different types of gastrointestinal disorders. Give three examples of a gastrointestinal disorder.

    a. _____
    b. _____
    c. _____

17. Gastroesophageal reflux disease (GERD) is defined as _____
    _____
    _____.

18. Antacids work to neutralize stomach acids. Give three situations in which antacids would be used to treat a GI disorder.

    a. _____
    b. _____
    c. _____

19. An ulcer is a _____ caused by _____ usually combined with _____.

20. An ulcer caused by stomach acids may also affect other structures, such as the _____ and the _____.

21. List three causes of ulcers.

    a. _____
    b. _____
    c. _____

QUESTIONS

Using what you have learned from the textbook, answer each question with one or two phrases or short sentences.

22. What is *Helicobacter pylori (H. pylori)*? _____
    _____

23. How is *Helicobacter pylori (H. pylori)* treated? _____
    _____

24. Inflammatory bowel disease is a chronic condition of the gastrointestinal tract. What are two types of inflammatory bowel disease?

    a. _____
    b. _____

25. What are four signs and symptoms of inflammatory bowel disease?

   a. _____
   b. _____
   c. _____
   d. _____

COMPLETION

Complete the following statements by filling in the blanks.

26. The medication of choice for inflammatory bowel disease are _____.

27. When the cause of diarrhea is unknown, it is beneficial to treat the symptom. List two reasons why it is beneficial to treat the symptom of diarrhea.

   a. _____
   b. _____

28. List the three ways in which antidiarrhea medications works.

   a. _____
   b. _____
   c. _____

29. When are antiflatulents used?

   a. _____
   b. _____

30. Laxatives are medications used to _____, to _____, and to _____.

31. There are times when a laxative should not be used to treat a GI disorder. List four contraindications for laxatives.

   a. _____
   b. _____
   c. _____
   d. _____

QUESTIONS

Using what you have learned from the textbook, answer each question with one or two phrases or short sentences.

32. Laxatives are used to relieve constipation and assist in the passing of feces through the lower GI tract. Some individuals abuse laxatives the same way that individuals can abuse other substances. What is the result of laxative abuse?

   _____
   _____

33. What is the difference between an antiemetic and an emetic medication?
   _____
   _____

34. There are circumstances when emetics may cause harm and should not be used. What are three circumstances during which emetics should not be used?
   a. _____
   b. _____
   c. _____

35. What is the name of a common OTC emetic that will usually cause vomiting within 20 minutes? _____

SUMMARY

The GI system can be affected by many different disorders. Most or all of these disorders, GI disorders, may cause significant discomfort in the body. They may also affect an individual's nutritional intake, which may then cause additional health problems. A basic understanding of these illnesses and the medications used to treat them will help the UAP to administer gastrointestinal medications safely and effectively.

Chapter 24
Medications for Treating Musculoskeletal Disorders

Learning Objectives

After completing the exercises in this chapter, you should be able to:

1. Spell and define terms.
2. Discuss the uses, adverse reactions, and special considerations for various medications used to treat musculoskeletal system disorders.

INTRODUCTION

The exercises you complete in this chapter will address the following key concepts from the textbook chapter:

- various disorders of the musculoskeletal system
- medications used to treat various disorders of the musculoskeletal system

VOCABULARY

Define the following terms.

1. inflammation _____
2. spondylitis _____
3. muscle spasms _____
4. peritonitis _____
5. myasthenia gravis _____

COMPLETION

Complete the following statements by filling in the blanks.

6. The musculoskeletal system gives the body _____ and the _____.

7. Disorders of the musculoskeletal system primarily include _____ and _____ of joints and muscles along with disorders that impact _____.

8. List four conditions skeletal muscle relaxants are used to treat.

    a. _____
    b. _____
    c. _____
    d. _____

9. The muscle stimulant, anticholinesterase (Prostigmin), is used to treat symptoms of _____.

10. Inflammation is a protective response of the body to _____ or _____. Inflammation may be _____ or _____.

11. List four symptoms of inflammation.

    a. _____
    b. _____
    c. _____
    d. _____

12. List five disorders that are treated with anti-inflammatory medications.
    a. _____
    b. _____
    c. _____
    d. _____
    e. _____

QUESTIONS

Using what you have learned from the textbook, answer each question with one or two phrases or short sentences.

13. What do anti-inflammatory medications do?
    _____
    _____

14. Nonsteroidal anti-inflammatory medications (NSAIDs) may cause bleeding. What are five signs and symptoms of bleeding?
    a. _____
    b. _____
    c. _____
    d. _____
    e. _____

15. Celebrex is a COX-2 inhibitor. What benefits does Celebrex have over nonsteroidal anti-inflammatory medications (NSAIDs)?
    a. _____
    b. _____

16. Disease-modifying antirheumatic medications (DMARDs) are used to treat rheumatoid arthritis. What do these medications do?
    _____
    _____

17. What is gout? _____
    _____

18. What joints are affected by gout? _____
    _____

COMPLETION

Complete the following statements by filling in the blanks.

19. Treatment of acute symptoms of gout usually includes _____ and _____.

20. An individual with gout should follow a diet low in _____.

21. Osteoporosis is defined as _____.

22. Osteoporosis results in an increase in fractures, especially of the _____, _____, and _____.

23. Osteoporosis occurs most often in _____, _____ _____, and _____ (Myers, 2006).

SUMMARY

Musculoskeletal disorders may vary from joint pain and inflammation to great difficulty in moving or the inability to move. A basic understanding of these illnesses and the medications used to treat them will help the UAP to administer musculoskeletal medications safely and effectively to individuals suffering from these disorders.

Chapter 25
Medications for Treating Respiratory Disorders

Learning Objectives

After completing the exercises in this chapter, you should be able to:
1. Spell and define terms.
2. Identify causes of respiratory disorders.
3. Discuss the uses, adverse reactions, and special considerations for various respiratory medications.

INTRODUCTION

The exercises you complete in this chapter will address the following key concepts from the textbook chapter:

- common causes of various respiratory disorders
- medications used to treat various respiratory disorders

VOCABULARY

Define the following terms.

1. bronchitis _____
2. allergy _____
3. epigastric distress _____
4. rebound nasal congestion _____
5. asthma _____
6. emphysema _____

MATCHING

There are many different types of respiratory medications. Each medication treats different symptoms or treats them in a different way. Draw lines to connect the type of medication on the left with the description of what it does in the right column.

7. decongestants
8. antihistamines
9. antitussives
10. expectorants
11. bronchodilators
12. corticosteroids
13. antileukotrienes
14. cromolyn sodium
15. smoking cessation products

a. used for the prevention, treatment, and management of asthma
b. relieve spasms in the air passages of the lungs and increase the aeration of the lungs
c. used for prevention of asthma attacks including the prevention of bronchospasms brought on by exercise
d. relieve allergy symptoms
e. aid individuals in quitting smoking
f. help loosen mucus, liquefy bronchial secretions, and remove phlegm (sputum)
g. used to treat asthma and COPD
h. prevents coughing in an individual who does not need to cough
i. relieve symptoms of nasal congestion

COMPLETION

Complete the following statements by filling in the blanks.

16. Respiratory disorders may be caused by many different factors. List three causes of respiratory disorders.

    a. _____
    b. _____
    c. _____

17. Decongestants are used to provide relief of nasal congestion. List three situations in which a decongestant would be used to treat nasal congestion.

    a. _____
    b. _____
    c. _____

18. Antihistamines are used to treat allergy symptoms caused by many different allergens. List three allergy symptoms treated by an antihistamine.

    a. _____
    b. _____
    c. _____

QUESTIONS

Using what you have learned from the textbook, answer each question with one or two phrases or short sentences.

19. What are the two categories of antitussive medication?

    a. _____
    b. _____

20. What are the three categories of bronchodilators?

    a. _____
    b. _____
    c. _____

21. What respiratory disorders may be treated with the use of bronchodilators?

    a. _____
    b. _____
    c. _____

22. By what two routes is cromolyn sodium administered?

    a. _____
    b. _____

COMPLETION

Complete the following statements by filling in the blanks.

23. Cigarette smoking accounts for over ___% of all cancer deaths, including ___ percent of lung cancer deaths. Cigarette smoking is also responsible for _____ _____, _____ and _____ _____ _____, _____, and _____.

24. Smoking cessation may be aided by the use of _____, _____, _____, _____, or _____ _____.

SUMMARY

Respiratory disorders may range from the common cold to allergies and asthma to pneumonia. It is the UAP's responsibility to have a basic understanding of these illnesses and the medications used to treat them. This understanding will help the UAP to administer medications safely and effectively to individuals with respiratory disorders.

Chapter 26
Medications for Treating Urinary Disorders

Learning Objectives

After completing the exercises in this chapter, you should be able to:

1. Spell and define terms.
2. Discuss the uses, adverse reactions, and special considerations for various genitourinary tract medications.

INTRODUCTION

The exercises you complete in this chapter will address the following key concepts from the textbook chapter:

- common causes of various urinary disorder
- various medications used to treat disorders of the urinary system

VOCABULARY

Define the following terms.

1. BPH _____
2. nocturia _____
3. edema _____
4. diuresis _____
5. hyperkalemia _____
6. cystitis _____
7. ascites _____
8. stomatitis _____

MATCHING

There are many different types of urinary medications. Each medication treats different symptoms or treats them in a different way. Draw lines to connect the type of medication on the left with the description of what it does in the right column.

9. diuretics
10. urinary system antibacterials
11. urinary system anti-infectives
12. antispasmodics
13. cholinergics
14. urinary analgesics
15. medications to treat benign prostatic hypertrophy

a. treat urinary tract infections
b. prevent spasms of the urinary bladder
c. treat acute and chronic upper and lower urinary tract infections.
d. treat the burning, pain, discomfort, and urinary urgency
e. increase urine output and relieve or prevent edema
f. treat benign prostatic hypertrophy (BPH)
g. treat nonobstructive urinary retention

COMPLETION

Complete the following statements by filling in the blanks.

16. The urinary system is responsible for _____, _____, and _____.

17. The urinary system is made up of the _____, the _____, the _____, and the _____.

18. List three disorders of the urinary system.

   a. _____

   b. _____

   c. _____

QUESTIONS

Using what you have learned from the textbook, answer each question with one or two phrases or short sentences.

19. The administration of a diuretic requires the UAP to give special care to an individual. Regardless of what type of diuretic the UAP is administering, what two things should a UAP do for an individual every day?

   a. _____

   b. _____

20. What type of diuretic is administered in acute care settings *only* by licensed health care providers?

   _____

21. When an individual is taking a certain type of diuretic called a potassium-sparing diuretic, he may experience hyperkalemia. Hyperkalemia is a high level of potassium in the blood. What are three symptoms of hyperkalemia?

   a. _____

   b. _____

   c. _____

22. Antispasmodics prevent spasms of the urinary bladder. What symptoms are relieved when bladder spasms are prevented?

   a. _____

   b. _____

   c. _____

23. Benign prostatic hypertrophy (BPH) is most common in men over 50 years of age. What are the signs and symptoms of BPH?

   a. _____

   b. _____

   c. _____

   d. _____

   e. _____

24. Why must the UAP wear gloves when handling and administering antiandrogens?

   _____

25. Some types of medications will discolor an individual's urine. Where would a UAP go to find information on medications and the effects they would have on an individual's body?

_____
_____
_____

SUMMARY

Urinary disorders may cause discomfort for the individual who experiences them. It is important for the UAP to observe and report any unusual symptoms that may indicate a kidney or urinary tract disorder to the individual's licensed health care provider. A basic understanding of these illnesses and the medications used to treat them will help the UAP to administer urinary medications safely and effectively.

Chapter 27
Medications for Treating Reproductive System Disorders

Learning Objectives

After completing the exercises in this chapter, you should be able to:

1. Spell and define terms.
2. Discuss the uses, adverse reactions, and special considerations for various medications used to treat reproductive system disorders.
3. State four possible causes of erectile dysfunction.
4. State the risks and benefits of hormone replacement therapy.

INTRODUCTION

The exercises you complete in this chapter will address the following key concepts from the textbook chapter:

- various medications used to treat disorders of the reproductive system
- potential causes of erectile dysfunction in men
- hormone replacement therapy with risks and benefits

VOCABULARY

Define the following terms.

1. menopause _____
2. HRT _____
3. hirsutism _____
4. amenorrhea _____
5. erectile dysfunction _____
6. hypercalcemia _____

COMPLETION

Complete the following statements by filling in the blanks.

7. Reproductive system structures in women include the _____, _____, and _____.

8. Reproductive system structures in men include the _____, _____, and _____.

9. Disorders of the reproductive system may include _____, _____, and _____.

10. Hormone replacement therapy (HRT) medications are used to replace or maintain a level of _____ and/or _____ that a woman's body has _____.

11. Oral contraceptives are medications used to _____.

12. Erectile dysfunction, also called impotence, may be caused by many different factors. List four of the factors that may cause erectile dysfunction.

    a. _____
    b. _____
    c. _____
    d. _____

13. Viagra is a medication used to treat erectile dysfunction. Individuals who are already at risk of cardiac disorders may experience significant cardiovascular events when taking Viagra. List three possible cardiovascular events that may occur.

    a. _____

    b. _____

    c. _____

QUESTIONS

Using what you have learned from the textbook, answer each question with one or two phrases or short sentences.

14. What is estrogen used for? _____
    _____
    _____

15. What are progestins used for? _____
    _____
    _____

16. What are testosterones used for in males? _____
    _____
    _____

17. What are testosterones used for in females? _____
    _____
    _____

18. What are the benefits of hormone replacement therapy (HRT)? _____
    _____
    _____

19. What are the risks of HRT? _____
    _____
    _____

20. Although oral contraceptives are usually safe for women, there are certain women who should *not* take oral contraceptives because of past or present medical history. What are three medical issues that would make oral contraceptive use unsafe for a woman?

    a. _____

    b. _____

    c. _____

SUMMARY

Disorders of the reproductive system may range from structural disorders to sexual disorders. A basic understanding of these illnesses and the medications used to treat them will help the UAP to administer these medications safely and effectively to those who are dealing with disorders of the reproductive system.

MODULE 5
COMMUNICATION AND DOCUMENTATION

Chapter 28
Role of the Unlicensed Assistive Personnel (UAP) in Medication Administration

Learning Objectives

After completing the exercises in this chapter, you should be able to:

1. Spell and define terms.
2. Explain the role of the UAP in medication administration.
3. List the key ingredients of a good relationship.
4. Briefly describe the communication process.
5. List five possible barriers to effective listening and communication.
6. List the four senses used in medication administration.
7. Describe the difference between subjective observation and objective observation.
8. Briefly describe three possible objective observations for each of the body's systems.
9. List the four questions that must be answered in order to report effectively.
10. Provide three examples of an emergency situation.
11. Provide three examples of a nonemergency situation.
12. Describe two situations when verbal reports are used to communicate with others.
13. State two pieces of information that should be included in a written report.
14. List ten guidelines for charting.

INTRODUCTION

The exercises you complete in this chapter will address the following key concepts from the textbook chapter:

- the role of the UAP in medication administration
- the key ingredients of a good relationship
- the communication process
- the difference between subjective observation and objective observation
- how to report effectively
- emergency and nonemergency situations
- verbal reports
- written reports
- guidelines for charting

VOCABULARY

Define the following terms.

1. licensed health care providers _____

2. administer _____
3. assessment _____
4. observation _____
5. objective observation _____
6. subjective observation _____
7. communication book _____
8. wheezing _____
9. body language _____
10. aphasia _____

COMPLETION

Complete the following statements by filling in the blanks.

11. When performing the task of medication administration, the UAP follows the instructions of a _____.

12. If the UAP notices a change in an individual's condition, he should immediately _____ the changes to the _____ and/or to the UAP's _____.

13. The UAP does not make an _____, an _____, or determine the _____ on the effect of a medication.

14. Changes in a medication order are made only by a _____.

Chapter 28 Role of the Unlicensed Assistive Personnel (UAP) in Medication Administration

QUESTIONS

Using what you have learned from the textbook, answer each question with one or two phrases or short sentences.

15. Why is the UAP an important member of the health care team?

    _____

16. What information can the UAP bring to the rest of the health care team?

    _____

17. Besides giving safe and effective daily care, how can the UAP have a positive effect on an individual's medical care? _____

    _____

18. Why are good relationships important? _____

    _____

19. Why is trust important when caring for individuals? _____

    _____

20. What are the three main ways communication occurs?
    a. _____
    b. _____
    c. _____

21. What is needed to communicate effectively?
    a. _____
    b. _____

22. What does the UAP use to make an observation about an individual's condition?

    _____

23. What sense would the UAP be using if he sees an individual trip and fall?

    _____

24. What sense would the UAP be using if he hears an individual crying?

    _____

25. What sense would the UAP be using if he smells a bad odor?

    _____

26. What sense would the UAP be using if he feels that an individual's skin is clammy?

    _____

LISTS

Using what you have learned from the textbook, complete the following lists.

27. Give two examples of objective observations that are not listed in the textbook.
    a. _____
    b. _____

28. Give two examples of subjective observations that are not listed in the textbook.

    a. _____

    b. _____

29. List three important criteria for observations made by the UAP.

    a. _____

    b. _____

    c. _____

30. List five barriers to effective communication.

    a. _____

    b. _____

    c. _____

    d. _____

    e. _____

CHOICES

For the statements below, place an "S" after the subjective observation or an "O" after the objective observation.

31. Mary is acting funny this morning. _____

32. Mary did not eat breakfast this morning. _____

33. Sam slept for four hours before waking up at 2 a.m. _____

34. Sam behaved badly at dinner tonight. _____

35. Judy acted out after lunch today, yelling and banging the table for at least five minutes.

    _____

36. Judy was being goofy this morning and called me some bad names.

    _____

37. Mark took his medication at 4 p.m. At 4:08 p.m., he began to complain of a headache.

    _____

MATCHING

The human body can be thought of as a set of systems, each system doing its own job to help the body function properly. On the left is a list of body systems. Draw a line to connect each body system in the left column with its description in the right column.

38. integumentary system   a. brain, spinal cord, and nerves

39. musculoskeletal system   b. glands

40. cardiovascular system   c. mouth, teeth, throat, esophagus, stomach, large and small intestines, gallbladder, liver, and pancreas

41. respiratory system

42. nervous system   d. heart, blood vessels, and blood

43. senses
44. urinary system
45. gastrointestinal system
46. endocrine system
47. reproductive system

e. skin and nails
f. breast, vagina, ovaries, testes, penis
g. muscles, bones, and joints
h. eyes, ears, nose, sense of touch
i. kidneys, ureters, bladder, and urethra
j. nose, throat, trachea, bronchi, and lungs

COMPLETION

Complete the following statements by filling in the blanks.

48. List the four things a UAP must know in order to report effectively.
    a. _____
    b. _____
    c. _____
    d. _____

49. When the UAP notices a change in an individual's condition, it is the UAP's responsibility to _____, _____, and _____.

50. It is not the UAP's responsibility to _____ or _____ the changes he observes.

51. List three examples of an emergency situation.
    a. _____
    b. _____
    c. _____

52. In an emergency situation, the UAP should _____.

53. In an emergency, if a UAP is working with other staff members, he should _____.

54. In an emergency, if the UAP is working alone, he should _____.

55. If the UAP is trained in first aid, he should _____.

56. After the individual is out of immediate danger, the UAP would do two tasks. List the two tasks the UAP would do.
    a. _____
    b. _____

57. List three examples of a nonemergency situation.

    a. _____

    b. _____

    c. _____

58. If a nonemergency situation occurs during the night, it may be reasonable to _____.

59. To find the specific time period required to report a nonemergency situation, the UAP should refer to _____.

QUESTIONS

Using what you have learned from the textbook, answer each question with one or two phrases or short sentences.

60. What is the difference between a verbal report and a written report? _____

61. List three occasions when a UAP would use a verbal report to communicate with another staff member.

    a. _____

    b. _____

    c. _____

62. How would the UAP report a subjective observation? Give an example of reporting a subjective observation that is not in the textbook. _____

63. How would the UAP report an objective observation? Give an example of reporting an objective observation that is not in the textbook. _____

64. What are the three things a UAP should report at the end of his shift?

    a. _____

    b. _____

    c. _____

65. What is the difference between a communication book (a logbook) and an individual's record? _____

66. What six pieces of information should be included in an individual's record and in the communication book?

   a. _____
   b. _____
   c. _____
   d. _____
   e. _____
   f. _____

67. When charting or documenting in an individual's medical record, is it okay to use a pencil? If not, what must you use? _____

68. Is it okay to erase or to use correction fluid like Wite Out®? _____

69. If not, how do you correct an error? _____

70. Is it okay to chart for your friend or to chart all of your tasks at the beginning of your shift? If not, why not? _____

71. Regarding question 70, when should charting be done? _____

72. Following is a table of standard and international times. Fill in the empty squares with the correct standard clock or international (Int'l) times.

International Time

STANDARD CLOCK	INT'L. TIME	STANDARD CLOCK	INT'L. TIME
a.m. 12 midnight	2400	p.m.	1200
1		1	
	0200		1400
3	0300		1500
4		4	
5		5	1700
6	0600	6	
	0700	7	
		8	2000
9			2100
10			
11			2300

(Delmar/Cengage Learning)

73. How do you indicate minutes using international time? _____
_____

74. Write the following times using international time.

   a. 1:25 a.m. _____
   b. 3:17 p.m. _____
   c. 7:42 a.m. _____
   d. 4:30 p.m. _____
   e. 10:15 a.m. _____
   f. 9:05 p.m. _____

SUMMARY

The role of the UAP is to observe, record, and report. Developing good observation skills; knowing when, how, to whom, and what to report; and documenting in a clear and concise manner are all skills that a UAP must practice in order to provide safe and effective care. Licensed health care providers depend on the UAP and the information he brings to them to provide quality care.

Chapter 29
Transcription of Licensed Health Care Provider Orders

Learning Objectives

After completing the exercises in this chapter, you should be able to:
1. Spell and define terms.
2. Explain the importance of accurate and complete documentation and transcription.
3. List the seven general principles of documentation and transcription.
4. Transcribe licensed health care providers' orders onto a medication sheet for a liquid form of medication and a solid form of medication.
5. Document medication administration onto an individual's medication sheet.
6. Write a progress note.
7. Discontinue a medication on a medication sheet.
8. Post and verify a transcribed order.
9. Complete a monthly quality review.

INTRODUCTION

The exercises you complete in this chapter will address the following key concepts from the textbook chapter:

- transcription
- documentation
- posting and verification
- monthly quality review

VOCABULARY

Define the following terms.

1. transcribe _____
2. medication sheet _____
3. start date _____
4. stop date _____
5. discontinuing _____
6. medication progress note _____
7. posting _____
8. verifying _____
9. monthly quality review _____

COMPLETION

Complete the following statements by filling in the blanks.

10. It is very important that information is transcribed accurately and completely onto the appropriate documents. Accurate and complete transcription is essential for three reasons. List the three reasons below:

    a. _____
    b. _____
    c. _____

11. There are seven general principles or guidelines that must be followed whenever documentation or transcription is completed. These guidelines help staff to provide accuracy and thorough completion. List the seven guidelines below:

    a. _____
    b. _____
    c. _____
    d. _____
    e. _____
    f. _____
    g. _____

12. Although different documents may be used from one work setting to another to track medication records, all documents must contain the following basic information:
    a. _____
    b. _____
    c. _____
    d. _____
    e. _____
    f. _____

13. On a medication sheet, each medication must have the following information listed:
    a. _____
    b. _____
    c. _____
    d. _____
    e. _____
    f. _____
    g. _____
    h. _____

CHOICES

14. From the list below, circle five types of licensed health care providers who can write a medication order.

nurse practitioner	clinical nurse specialist	physician's assistant
dentist	UAP	RN
receptionist	LPN	group home manager
physician		

INTERPRETATION

For the licensed HCP orders below, write each piece of information into the correct space. Note that brand names are given in parentheses.

15. Order: carbamazepine (Tegretol) 200 mg 2 tabs by mouth bid. Notify licensed HCP if seizure occurs.
    a. Generic name _____
    b. Brand name _____
    c. Strength of the medication _____
    d. Amount to be given _____
    e. Route _____
    f. Frequency _____
    g. Special instructions/precautions _____

16. Order: digoxin (Lanoxin) 0.25 mg 1 tab by mouth every day in a.m. Notify licensed HCP if resting pulse <60 bpm.

   a. Generic name _____
   b. Brand name _____
   c. Strength of the medication _____
   d. Amount to be given _____
   e. Route _____
   f. Frequency _____
   g. Special instructions/precautions _____

17. Order: erythromycin 333 mg 1 tab by mouth qid.

   a. Generic name _____
   b. Brand name _____
   c. Strength of the medication _____
   d. Amount to be given _____
   e. Route _____
   f. Frequency _____
   g. Special instructions/precautions _____

18. Order: sertraline (Zoloft) 50 mg 1 tab by mouth bid. Notify licensed HCP if individual demonstrates decreased appetite or sleeps >12 hrs/day.

   a. Generic name _____
   b. Brand name _____
   c. Strength of the medication _____
   d. Amount to be given _____
   e. Route _____
   f. Frequency _____
   g. Special instructions/precautions _____

19. Order: ibuprofen (Motrin) 100 mg 4 tabs by mouth tid. Notify licensed HCP if right knee is hot to touch or if individual c/o sharp pain on ambulation (when walking).

   a. Generic name _____
   b. Brand name _____
   c. Strength of the medication _____
   d. Amount to be given _____
   e. Route _____
   f. Frequency _____
   g. Special instructions/precautions _____

20. Order: alprazolam (Xanax) 2 mg 1 tab by mouth bid. Notify licensed HCP if individual c/o insomnia or tension headache.

   a. Generic name _____
   b. Brand name _____

c. Strength of the medication _____

d. Amount to be given _____

e. Route _____

f. Frequency _____

g. Special instructions/precautions _____

21. Order: dextromethorphan (Vicks Formula 44) 15 mg/5 mL 10 mL q6h by mouth WA.

   a. Generic name _____

   b. Brand name _____

   c. Strength of the medication _____

   d. Amount to be given _____

   e. Route _____

   f. Frequency _____

   g. Special instructions/precautions _____

22. Order: albuterol (Ventolin) 90 mcg/dose 2 inhalations by mouth 15 minutes before exercising. Do not exceed four doses in a 24-hour period.

   a. Generic name _____

   b. Brand name _____

   c. Strength of the medication _____

   d. Amount to be given _____

   e. Route _____

   f. Frequency _____

   g. Special instructions/precautions _____

23. Order: guaifenesin and codeine (Robitussin A-C) 10 mg/5 mL 2 tsp by mouth q6h WA.

   a. Generic name _____

   b. Brand name _____

   c. Strength of the medication _____

   d. Amount to be given _____

   e. Route _____

   f. Frequency _____

   g. Special instructions/precautions _____

24. Order: brompheniramine and phenylephrine (Dimetane Decongestant Elixir) 5 mg/5 mL 2 tsp by mouth q4h. Notify licensed HCP if symptoms continue for >3 days.

   a. Generic name _____

   b. Brand name _____

   c. Strength of the medication _____

   d. Amount to be given _____

   e. Route _____

   f. Frequency _____

   g. Special instructions/precautions _____

TRANSCRIBING A MEDICATION ORDER

In the charts that follow, transcribe the information from the following licensed HCP orders onto the medication sheets. Note that brand names are given in parentheses. Include start date and stop dates, if given, along with times that the medication is to be given.

25. Order reads: fluconazole (Diflucan) 150 mg 1 tab by mouth once in a.m. Notify licensed HCP if individual c/o vaginal itching or irritation. Order is dated 12/3/09.

Medication or Treatment		Hour	1	2	3	4	5	6	7	8	9	10	11	12	13	14	15	16	17	18	19	20	21	22	23	24	25	26	27	28	29	30	31
Start	Generic																																	
	Brand																																	
Stop	Strength																																	
	Amount																																	
	Frequency																																	
	Route																																	
Special Instructions/Precautions																																		

(Delmar/Cengage Learning)

26. Order reads: chlorpromazine (Thorazine) 10 mg 1 tab by mouth q6h × 3 days. Notify licensed HCP if vomiting continues after med is given. Order is dated 10/25/09.

Medication or Treatment		Hour	1	2	3	4	5	6	7	8	9	10	11	12	13	14	15	16	17	18	19	20	21	22	23	24	25	26	27	28	29	30	31
Start	Generic																																	
	Brand																																	
Stop	Strength																																	
	Amount																																	
	Frequency																																	
	Route																																	
Special Instructions/Precautions																																		

(Delmar/Cengage Learning)

27. Order reads: penicillin V potassium (Penicillin VK) oral suspension 250 mg by mouth tid × 10 days. Order is dated 5/21/10. Pharmacy label directions include: Take 2 teaspoons (10 cc) by mouth 3 times a day for 10 days. Shake well before pouring.

Medication or Treatment	Hour	1	2	3	4	5	6	7	8	9	10	11	12	13	14	15	16	17	18	19	20	21	22	23	24	25	26	27	28	29	30	31
Start Generic																																	
Brand																																	
Stop Strength																																	
Amount																																	
Frequency																																	
Route																																	
Special Instructions/Precautions																																	

(Delmar/Cengage Learning)

28. Order reads: guaifenesin and codeine (Robitussin AC) 10 mL by mouth q6h WA × 3 days. Notify licensed HCP's office to schedule follow-up visit for 9/27/11. Order is dated 9/23/11. Pharmacy label directions state: Take 2 t (10 cc) by mouth every 6 hours while awake for 3 days.

Medication or Treatment	Hour	1	2	3	4	5	6	7	8	9	10	11	12	13	14	15	16	17	18	19	20	21	22	23	24	25	26	27	28	29	30	31
Start Generic																																	
Brand																																	
Stop Strength																																	
Amount																																	
Frequency																																	
Route																																	
Special Instructions/Precautions																																	

(Delmar/Cengage Learning)

DOCUMENTING A MEDICATION GIVEN

In the charts that follow, transcribe the licensed HCP order onto the medication sheet. Include the start date in each order. Set up the documentation to begin giving the medication on the start date. Include the stop date if given. Initial the medication block to indicate that the first dose of medication has been given. Write your name and initials in the signature section.

29. Order reads: diphenhydramine (Benadryl) 50 mg 1 tab by mouth q6h × 10 days. Notify licensed HCP if rash continues after 7 days. Order is written at 11 a.m. By the time you return to your work site, you will be able to give the first dose at 1 p.m. Order is dated 7/6/10.

Medication or Treatment		Hour	1	2	3	4	5	6	7	8	9	10	11	12	13	14	15	16	17	18	19	20	21	22	23	24	25	26	27	28	29	30	31
Start	Generic																																	
	Brand																																	
Stop	Strength Amount																																	
	Frequency Route																																	
Special Instructions/Precautions																																		

Signature	Initials	Signature	Initials	Signature	Initials

(Delmar/Cengage Learning)

30. Order reads: tetracycline 250 mg 1 tab by mouth q6h × 10 days. May be taken with food if individual c/o nausea. Order is written at 4:30 p.m. By the time you return to your work site, you will be able to give the first dose at 6 p.m. Order is dated 8/2/11.

Medication or Treatment		Hour	1	2	3	4	5	6	7	8	9	10	11	12	13	14	15	16	17	18	19	20	21	22	23	24	25	26	27	28	29	30	31
Start	Generic																																	
	Brand																																	
Stop	Strength Amount																																	
	Frequency Route																																	
Special Instructions/Precautions																																		

Signature	Initials	Signature	Initials	Signature	Initials

(Delmar/Cengage Learning)

31. Order reads: cimetidine (Tagamet) 400 mg 2 tabs by mouth at bedtime. Notify licensed HCP if individual c/o abdominal pain or heartburn. Order is written at 1:30 p.m. You will be able to give the first dose at bedtime. Order is dated 4/7/09.

Medication or Treatment		Hour	1	2	3	4	5	6	7	8	9	10	11	12	13	14	15	16	17	18	19	20	21	22	23	24	25	26	27	28	29	30	31
Start	Generic																																	
	Brand																																	
Stop	Strength Amount																																	
	Frequency Route																																	
Special Instructions/Precautions																																		
Signature				Initials	Signature								Initials	Signature															Initials				

(Delmar/Cengage Learning)

32. Order reads: docusate sodium (Colace) 100 mg 2 tabs by mouth bid. Give with 8 oz. water. Order is written at 9:30 a.m. By the time you return to your work site, you will be able to give the first dose after 11 a.m. Order is dated 5/1/10.

Medication or Treatment		Hour	1	2	3	4	5	6	7	8	9	10	11	12	13	14	15	16	17	18	19	20	21	22	23	24	25	26	27	28	29	30	31
Start	Generic																																	
	Brand																																	
Stop	Strength Amount																																	
	Frequency Route																																	
Special Instructions/Precautions																																		
Signature				Initials	Signature								Initials	Signature															Initials				

(Delmar/Cengage Learning)

33. Order reads: ibuprofen (Motrin) 200 mg 1 tab by mouth q6h prn for T > 101°F. Notify licensed HCP if fever lasts for more than 24 hours. Order is written at 2:30 p.m. By the time you return to your work site, you will be able to give the first dose at 4 p.m. Order is dated 3/6/10.

Medication or Treatment		Hour	1	2	3	4	5	6	7	8	9	10	11	12	13	14	15	16	17	18	19	20	21	22	23	24	25	26	27	28	29	30	31
Start	Generic																																	
	Brand																																	
Stop	Strength																																	
	Amount																																	
	Frequency																																	
	Route																																	
Special Instructions/Precautions																																		

Signature	Initials	Signature	Initials	Signature	Initials

(Delmar/Cengage Learning)

DISCONTINUING A MEDICATION ORDER

In the charts that follow, complete the documentation to show that a medication has been discontinued. Initials are included in the chart for each time the medication was given. Write your name and initials in the signature section.

34. Order reads: chlorpromazine (Thorazine) 10 mg 1 tab by mouth q6h × 3 days. Notify licensed HCP if vomiting continues after medication is given. Order is dated 10/04/09. The first dose was given on 10/4/09 at 12 p.m. The individual continues to vomit. The UAP notifies the licensed HCP. On 10/5/09 at 8 a.m. the licensed HCP orders the medication discontinued. Discontinue the medication on the chart that follows.

Medication or Treatment		Hour	1	2	3	4	5	6	7	8	9	10	11	12	13	14	15	16	17	18	19	20	21	22	23	24	25	26	27	28	29	30	31
Start 10/04/09	Generic chlorpromazine	12 AM	x	x	x	x	CJ		x	x	x	x	x	x	x	x	x	x	x	x	x	x	x	x	x	x	x	x	x	x	x	x	x
	Brand Thorazine	6 AM	x	x	x	x	CJ		x	x	x	x	x	x	x	x	x	x	x	x	x	x	x	x	x	x	x	x	x	x	x	x	x
Stop	Strength 10 mg																																	
	Amount 1 tab	12 PM	x	x	x	PL		x	x	x	x	x	x	x	x	x	x	x	x	x	x	x	x	x	x	x	x	x	x	x	x	x	
	Frequency q6h																																	
	Route By mouth	6 PM	x	x	x	RT		x	x	x	x	x	x	x	x	x	x	x	x	x	x	x	x	x	x	x	x	x	x	x	x	x	
Special Instructions/Precautions Notify Licensed HCP If vomiting continues after medication is given.																																		

Signature	Initials	Signature	Initials	Signature	Initials
Paul Leonard	PL	Cynthia Jaccaboni	CJ		
Ronald Tuttle	RT				

(Delmar/Cengage Learning)

35. Order reads: tetracycline 250 mg 1 tab by mouth q6h × 10 days. May be taken with food if individual c/o nausea. Order is dated 8/1/11. The first dose was given on 8/1/11 at 10 a.m. On 8/3/11 the individual develops a rash. The licensed HCP discontinues the medication on 8/3/11 at 2 p.m. Discontinue the medication on the chart that follows.

Medication or Treatment		Hour	1	2	3	4	5	6	7	8	9	10	11	12	13	14	15	16	17	18	19	20	21	22	23	24	25	26	27	28	29	30	31
Start 8/1/11	Generic tetracycline	10 AM	PL	PL	PL								x	x	x	x	x	x	x	x	x	x	x	x	x	x	x	x	x	x	x	x	x
	Brand																																	
		4 AM	CR	CR									x	x	x	x	x	x	x	x	x	x	x	x	x	x	x	x	x	x	x	x	x
Stop	Strength 250 mg																																	
	Amount 1 tab	10 AM	CR	CR									x	x	x	x	x	x	x	x	x	x	x	x	x	x	x	x	x	x	x	x	x
	Frequency q6h																																	
	Route By mouth	4 PM	ST	ST									x	x	x	x	x	x	x	x	x	x	x	x	x	x	x	x	x	x	x	x	x
Special Instructions/Precautions May be taken with food if individual complains of nausea.																																	

Signature	Initials	Signature	Initials	Signature	Initials
Paul Leonard	PL	Sarah Thames	ST		
Charles Ridley	CR				

(Delmar/Cengage Learning)

36. Order reads: D/c Premarin 0.625 mg after 6/8/10. Notify licensed HCP if individual c/o hot flashes or vaginal dryness. Order is dated 6/3/10. Discontinue the medication on the following chart.

Medication or Treatment		Hour	1	2	3	4	5	6	7	8	9	10	11	12	13	14	15	16	17	18	19	20	21	22	23	24	25	26	27	28	29	30	31
Start 3/1/10	Generic estrogen																																	
	Brand Premarin	12 AM	PD	PD	PD																													
Stop	Strength 0.625 mg																																	
	Amount 1 tab																																	
	Frequency daily																																	
	Route by mouth																																	
Special Instructions/Precautions Notify licensed HCP if individual complains of hot flashes or vaginal dryness.																																	

Signature	Initials	Signature	Initials	Signature	Initials
Paul Dufresne	PD				

(Delmar/Cengage Learning)

37. Order reads: D/c Colace 100 mg bid. Begin senna (Senokot) 374 mg 1 tab by mouth at bedtime. Notify licensed HCP if BM does not occur in 3 days. Order is dated 7/7/10. Initials are included in the chart for each time the medication was given. Enter the stop date in the correct space and discontinue the medication. Begin a new chart for the new medication.

a.

Medication or Treatment		Hour	1	2	3	4	5	6	7	8	9	10	11	12	13	14	15	16	17	18	19	20	21	22	23	24	25	26	27	28	29	30	31
Start 6/25/10	Generic docusate sodium	8 AM	RB	RB	RB	RB	RB	RB	SL																									
	Brand Colace																																	
Stop 7/7/10	Strength 100 mg Amount 1 tab	4 PM	CT	CT	CT	CT	SL	SL																										
	Frequency bid Route By mouth																																	
Special Instructions/Precautions Notify HCP if BM does not occur in 3 days.																																		

Signature	Initials	Signature	Initials	Signature	Initials
Rodney Benson	RB	Samuel Livingston	SL		
Cynthia Turletto	CT				

b.

Medication or Treatment		Hour	1	2	3	4	5	6	7	8	9	10	11	12	13	14	15	16	17	18	19	20	21	22	23	24	25	26	27	28	29	30	31
Start 7/7/10	Generic senna																																	
	Brand Senokot																																	
Stop	Strength 374 mg Amount 1 tab	HS																																
	Frequency at bedtime Route By mouth																																	
Special Instructions/Precautions Notify licensed HCP if BM does not occur in 3 days.																																		

Signature	Initials	Signature	Initials	Signature	Initials

SPECIAL SITUATIONS

Some medication orders are given in unusual ways. In the charts below, show how a medication sheet would be set up to give a new medication that requires different dosages every day or smaller doses at first followed by larger doses after a certain period of time. Include times for giving the medication. Include start and stop dates if given. Sign the chart. Write in your initials as though you were giving the first dose.

38. Order reads: metoprolol (Lopressor) 50 mg 1 tab by mouth bid × 1 week, then 50 mg 1 tab by mouth tid × 1 week, then 50 mg 1 tab by mouth qid. Notify licensed HCP if individual c/o chest pains or SOB. The order is dated 3/14/11. Medication is to be started on 3/15/11.

  a. Week 1 chart:

Medication or Treatment		Hour	1	2	3	4	5	6	7	8	9	10	11	12	13	14	15	16	17	18	19	20	21	22	23	24	25	26	27	28	29	30	31
Start	Generic																																	
	Brand																																	
Stop	Strength																																	
	Amount																																	
	Frequency																																	
	Route																																	
Special Instructions/Precautions																																		
Signature				Initials		Signature								Initials		Signature													Initials					

(Delmar/Cengage Learning)

  b. Week 2 chart:

Medication or Treatment		Hour	1	2	3	4	5	6	7	8	9	10	11	12	13	14	15	16	17	18	19	20	21	22	23	24	25	26	27	28	29	30	31
Start	Generic																																	
	Brand																																	
Stop	Strength																																	
	Amount																																	
	Frequency																																	
	Route																																	
Special Instructions/Precautions																																		
Signature				Initials		Signature								Initials		Signature													Initials					

(Delmar/Cengage Learning)

c. Week 3 chart:

Medication or Treatment		Hour	1	2	3	4	5	6	7	8	9	10	11	12	13	14	15	16	17	18	19	20	21	22	23	24	25	26	27	28	29	30	31
Start	Generic																																	
	Brand																																	
Stop	Strength Amount Frequency Route																																	
Special Instructions/Precautions																																		
Signature					Initials	Signature								Initials	Signature													Initials					

(Delmar/Cengage Learning)

39. Order reads: sertraline (Zoloft) 50 mg 1 tab by mouth at bedtime × 1 week, then 100 mg 1 tab by mouth at bedtime × 1 week, then 150 mg 1 tab by mouth at bedtime. Notify licensed HCP if individual c/o dry mouth or decreased appetite. Order is dated 8/6/09.

a. Week 1 chart:

Medication or Treatment		Hour	1	2	3	4	5	6	7	8	9	10	11	12	13	14	15	16	17	18	19	20	21	22	23	24	25	26	27	28	29	30	31
Start	Generic																																	
	Brand																																	
Stop	Strength Amount Frequency Route																																	
Special Instructions/Precautions																																		
Signature					Initials	Signature								Initials	Signature													Initials					

(Delmar/Cengage Learning)

b. Week 2 chart:

Medication or Treatment		Hour	1	2	3	4	5	6	7	8	9	10	11	12	13	14	15	16	17	18	19	20	21	22	23	24	25	26	27	28	29	30	31
Start	Generic																																	
	Brand																																	
Stop	Strength Amount																																	
	Frequency Route																																	
Special Instructions/Precautions																																		
Signature						Initials	Signature										Initials	Signature													Initials			

(Delmar/Cengage Learning)

c. Week 3 chart:

Medication or Treatment		Hour	1	2	3	4	5	6	7	8	9	10	11	12	13	14	15	16	17	18	19	20	21	22	23	24	25	26	27	28	29	30	31
Start	Generic																																	
	Brand																																	
Stop	Strength Amount																																	
	Frequency Route																																	
Special Instructions/Precautions																																		
Signature						Initials	Signature										Initials	Signature													Initials			

(Delmar/Cengage Learning)

40. Original order reads: Dilantin 100 mg 1 tab by mouth qid. The licensed HCP is changing the anticonvulsant, Dilantin, to Depakene. To do so safely, the licensed HCP needs to decrease (titrate) the Dilantin and slowly begin and increase the new medication, Depakene. The licensed HCP order is dated 7/1/10. The licensed HCP order reads as follows:

Week 1: Decrease Dilantin to 100 mg 1 tab by mouth tid × 1 week.

Begin Depakene 250 mg 1 cap by mouth tid × 1 week.

Week 2: Decrease Dilantin to 100 mg 1 tab by mouth bid × 1 week.

Increase Depakene to 250 mg 1 cap by mouth qid × 1 week.

Week 3: D/c Dilantin.

Increase Depakene to 250 mg 2 caps by mouth bid.

Begin Depakene 250 mg 1 cap by mouth at bedtime × 1 week.

Week 4: Increase Depakene to 250 mg 2 caps by mouth bid plus

250 mg 2 caps by mouth at bedtime.

a. Week 1 charts:

Medication or Treatment		Hour	1	2	3	4	5	6	7	8	9	10	11	12	13	14	15	16	17	18	19	20	21	22	23	24	25	26	27	28	29	30	31
Start	Generic																																	
	Brand																																	
Stop	Strength Amount																																	
	Frequency Route																																	
Special Instructions/Precautions																																		
Signature				Initials	Signature							Initials		Signature													Initials						

(Delmar/Cengage Learning)

Medication or Treatment		Hour	1	2	3	4	5	6	7	8	9	10	11	12	13	14	15	16	17	18	19	20	21	22	23	24	25	26	27	28	29	30	31
Start	Generic																																	
	Brand																																	
Stop	Strength																																	
	Amount																																	
	Frequency																																	
	Route																																	
Special Instructions/Precautions																																		
Signature						Initials	Signature									Initials	Signature														Initials		

(Delmar/Cengage Learning)

b. Week 2 charts:

Medication or Treatment		Hour	1	2	3	4	5	6	7	8	9	10	11	12	13	14	15	16	17	18	19	20	21	22	23	24	25	26	27	28	29	30	31
Start	Generic																																	
	Brand																																	
Stop	Strength																																	
	Amount																																	
	Frequency																																	
	Route																																	
Special Instructions/Precautions																																		
Signature						Initials	Signature									Initials	Signature														Initials		

(Delmar/Cengage Learning)

Medication or Treatment		Hour	1	2	3	4	5	6	7	8	9	10	11	12	13	14	15	16	17	18	19	20	21	22	23	24	25	26	27	28	29	30	31
Start	Generic																																
	Brand																																
Stop	Strength Amount																																
	Frequency Route																																
Special Instructions/Precautions																																	

Signature		Initials	Signature		Initials	Signature		Initials

(Delmar/Cengage Learning)

c. Week 3 charts:

Medication or Treatment		Hour	1	2	3	4	5	6	7	8	9	10	11	12	13	14	15	16	17	18	19	20	21	22	23	24	25	26	27	28	29	30	31
Start	Generic																																
	Brand																																
Stop	Strength Amount																																
	Frequency Route																																
Special Instructions/Precautions																																	

Signature		Initials	Signature		Initials	Signature		Initials

(Delmar/Cengage Learning)

Medication or Treatment	Hour	1	2	3	4	5	6	7	8	9	10	11	12	13	14	15	16	17	18	19	20	21	22	23	24	25	26	27	28	29	30	31
Start — Generic																																
Brand																																
Stop — Strength / Amount / Frequency / Route																																

Special Instructions/Precautions

Signature		Initials	Signature		Initials	Signature		Initials

(Delmar/Cengage Learning)

d. Week 4 chart:

Medication or Treatment	Hour	1	2	3	4	5	6	7	8	9	10	11	12	13	14	15	16	17	18	19	20	21	22	23	24	25	26	27	28	29	30	31
Start — Generic																																
Brand																																
Stop — Strength / Amount / Frequency / Route																																

Special Instructions/Precautions

Signature		Initials	Signature		Initials	Signature		Initials

(Delmar/Cengage Learning)

Medication or Treatment	Hour	1	2	3	4	5	6	7	8	9	10	11	12	13	14	15	16	17	18	19	20	21	22	23	24	25	26	27	28	29	30	31
Start — Generic																																
Brand																																
Stop — Strength / Amount / Frequency / Route																																

Special Instructions/Precautions

Signature		Initials	Signature		Initials	Signature		Initials

(Delmar/Cengage Learning)

WRITING A PROGRESS NOTE

41. List three situations in which the UAP would have to write a progress note.

a. _____

b. _____

c. _____

In the charts that follow, write a progress note for each situation given.

42. Sam takes Zoloft 100 mg 1 tab by mouth bid. When you prepare his dose for 8 p.m., he states that he does not want to take it. When you ask him why, he says that he wants to stop taking his medication. He is feeling better. You explain that he feels better because of his medication. If he stops taking it, he may not continue to feel well. When you offer it again, he still refuses. You leave him and then reapproach after a few minutes. He still refuses to take his Zoloft.

Date	Time	Medication and Dosage	Held	Refused	Given	Reason	Result of Response	Signature

(Delmar/Cengage Learning)

43. Joyce takes Motrin prn for a fever greater than 101°F. When you approach her to give her usual medications at 4 p.m., you notice that she is withdrawn and looks ill. When you ask if she is okay, Joyce states that she feels "really hot." You put your hand on her forehead and she feels feverish. When you take her temperature, you see that she has a fever of 102.6°F.

Date	Time	Medication and Dosage	Held	Refused	Given	Reason	Result of Response	Signature

(Delmar/Cengage Learning)

44. David takes Ativan 2 mg 1 tab by mouth tid. When you go to prepare his 2 p.m. medications, you find that the last dose available was given at 8 a.m. The pharmacy has not yet delivered a new supply of Ativan for him.

Date	Time	Medication and Dosage	Held	Refused	Given	Reason	Result of Response	Signature

(Delmar/Cengage Learning)

45. Sarah takes Glucotrol, an antidiabetic medication, 10 mg 1 tab by mouth bid. You see a note in the communication book that Sarah's Glucotrol should not be given at 6 p.m. because she is having lab work done the following morning.

Date	Time	Medication and Dosage	Held	Refused	Given	Reason	Result of Response	Signature

(Delmar/Cengage Learning)

PRACTICAL APPLICATIONS
Performing Posting, Verification, and Monthly Quality Review

This section is completed as a team project. Your instructor will divide the class into teams. The project will then be completed as follows:

1. Each member of the team will transcribe and post orders from the licensed health care provider order form immediately following these instructions.
2. Once each team member has completed transcribing and posting the licensed HCP orders, team members will exchange their medication sheets and will verify each other's licensed HCP orders.
3. Once verification of the licensed HCP orders is completed, teams will then exchange their medication sheets with an alternate team.
4. Members of the alternate team will then complete a monthly quality review.

This section will give you a realistic practice in all three areas of posting, verification, and monthly quality review.

Here is the licensed health care provider order form with medications and treatments ordered (Figure 29-1). Transcribe and post the following orders onto the medication sheets provided.

				Mary Highlander DOB 4/16/1953 126 Main Street Westchester, IL 63506

Medical Center Hospital
Licensed Health Care Provider's Order Sheet
Instructions:
1. Imprint the individual's identification plate onto the form before placing form into the chart.
2. After each set of orders are written, remove the first yellow copy and send it to the pharmacy.
3. "X" out the remaining unused lines after the last yellow copy is used.

ALLERGIES   NKA

Date Ordered	Time Ordered	Posted	Verified	Use Ball Point Pen Only
12/1/09	10:00 AM			carbamazepine (Tegretol) 200 mg 2 tabs by mouth bid. Notify licensed HCP if seizure occurs. alprazolam (Xanax) 2 mg 1 tab by mouth bid. Notify licensed HCP if individual. c/o insomnia or tension headaches. Dimetane Decongestant Elixir 5 mg/5 mL 2 tsp by mouth q4h prn for congestion. Notify licensed HCP if symptoms continue for >3 days. Dr. James Proctor ~~~~
12/1/09	1:30 PM			cimetidine (Tagamet) 400 mg 2 tabs by mouth prn at bedtime for c/o heartburn. Position Mary in an upright position for at least 30 mins after meals for c/o heartburn. Dr. James Proctor ~~~~~~~~~~~~~~~~~~~~~~~~~~~~~

Figure 29-1 Sample Licensed Health Care Provider's Order Form used in an institutional setting *(Delmar/Cengage Learning)*

Medication or Treatment		Hour	1	2	3	4	5	6	7	8	9	10	11	12	13	14	15	16	17	18	19	20	21	22	23	24	25	26	27	28	29	30	31
Start	Generic																																
	Brand																																
Stop	Strength Amount																																
	Frequency Route																																
Special Instructions/Precautions																																	

Signature	Initials	Signature	Initials	Signature	Initials

(Delmar/Cengage Learning)

Medication or Treatment		Hour	1	2	3	4	5	6	7	8	9	10	11	12	13	14	15	16	17	18	19	20	21	22	23	24	25	26	27	28	29	30	31
Start	Generic																																
	Brand																																
Stop	Strength Amount																																
	Frequency Route																																
Special Instructions/Precautions																																	

Signature	Initials	Signature	Initials	Signature	Initials

(Delmar/Cengage Learning)

Medication or Treatment		Hour	1	2	3	4	5	6	7	8	9	10	11	12	13	14	15	16	17	18	19	20	21	22	23	24	25	26	27	28	29	30	31
Start	Generic																																	
	Brand																																	
Stop	Strength Amount																																	
	Frequency Route																																	
Special Instructions/Precautions																																		

Signature	Initials	Signature	Initials	Signature	Initials

(Delmar/Cengage Learning)

Medication or Treatment		Hour	1	2	3	4	5	6	7	8	9	10	11	12	13	14	15	16	17	18	19	20	21	22	23	24	25	26	27	28	29	30	31
Start	Generic																																	
	Brand																																	
Stop	Strength Amount																																	
	Frequency Route																																	
Special Instructions/Precautions																																		

Signature	Initials	Signature	Initials	Signature	Initials

(Delmar/Cengage Learning)

Medication or Treatment	Hour	1	2	3	4	5	6	7	8	9	10	11	12	13	14	15	16	17	18	19	20	21	22	23	24	25	26	27	28	29	30	31
Start — Generic																																
Brand																																
Stop — Strength / Amount																																
Frequency / Route																																
Special Instructions/Precautions																																

Signature	Initials	Signature	Initials	Signature	Initials

(Delmar/Cengage Learning)

Review the licensed HCP order form and the posted and verified orders on the previous pages. Use the review sheet provided (Figure 29-2) to complete your monthly quality review.

Monthly Review of Orders for _____ (month/year)
Patient/ Resident/ Client:_____

Medication or treatment	Date ordered	Licensed HCP	Transcription Date	Staff Member Transcribed	Accurate? Yes/No	Staff Member Reviewing

Action required? (yes/no) _____

If yes, state action plan:
_____
_____

Signature: _____

Figure 29-2 Sample Monthly Review Form *(Delmar/Cengage Learning)*

SUMMARY

As discussed in Chapters 5 and 28, effective communication is essential to safe and effective administration of medication. Transcription and medication progress notes, accurately completed, allow the UAP to communicate with coworkers and other members of the health care team. Posting and verification of orders and the completion of monthly quality reviews help to eliminate medication errors. The safety of the individual under the care of the UAP is protected.

MODULE 6
SAFETY

Chapter 30
Additional Considerations

Learning Objectives

After completing the exercises in this chapter, you should be able to:

1. Spell and define terms.
2. List the four guidelines for the administration of an over-the-counter medication.
3. Demonstrate the administration of an over-the-counter medication.
4. Name three types of medication interactions.
5. List five types of adverse medication effects.
6. Explain two ways to prevent adverse medication interactions.
7. Explain the difference between psychological dependence and physical dependence.
8. Explain the difference between hypersensitivity and anaphylactic reaction.
9. Describe the four processes that undergo change as an individual ages.
10. List the Six Wrongs of medication administration and give an example of each.
11. Explain the four guidelines to prevent misinterpretation of a licensed health care provider's order.
12. Describe the four steps to follow should a medication error occur.
13. Complete a medication occurrence form.
14. Complete a drug incident report.
15. List four reasons a medication refusal may occur.
16. Explain the difference between an active medication refusal and a passive medication refusal.
17. List four ways to deal with a medication refusal.

INTRODUCTION

The exercises you complete in this chapter will address the following key concepts from the textbook chapter:

- administration of an over-the-counter medication
- medication interactions and adverse effects
- medication dependence
- the aging process
- the Six Wrongs of medication administration
- medication reconciliation
- medication losses
- medication errors and refusals

VOCABULARY

Define the following terms.

1. medication interaction _____
2. adverse medication effects _____
3. anaphylactic reaction _____
4. cumulative effect of medications _____
5. the Gray List _____
6. the Six Wrongs _____
7. medication error _____
8. medication loss _____
9. medication reconciliation _____

QUESTIONS

Using what you have learned from the textbook, answer each question with one or two phrases or short sentences.

10. What must the UAP always remember about OTC medications? _____
_____

11. The textbook lists four guidelines to follow when handling OTC medications. What are the four guidelines?

   a. _____
   b. _____
   c. _____
   d. _____

12. What should the UAP do if he knows that an individual in his care is using alcohol, nicotine, caffeine, or any illegal drugs? _____
_____
_____

MATCHING

Draw lines connecting each term on the left with its description in the right column.

13. synergism
14. potentiation
15. antagonism
16. teratogenic effect
17. idiosyncrasy
18. tolerance
19. dependence
20. psychological dependence
21. physical dependence
22. hypersensitivity

a. one medication decreases or cancels out the effect of the other medication

b. one medication helps another for an effect that neither one could produce alone

c. one medication prolongs or multiplies the effect of the other medication

d. the body's cells actually have a need for the medication

e. an acquired need for a medication that may produce physical and/or psychological symptoms of withdrawal when the medication is discontinued

f. no physical withdrawal other than anxiety occurs when the medication is discontinued

g. an allergic response to a medication; may be of varying severity

h. administration of certain medications to pregnant women causes birth defects in newborns

i. a decreased response to a medication that develops over time after repeated doses are given

j. a unique, unusual response to a medication

COMPLETION

Complete the following statements by filling in the blanks.

23. Anaphylactic reaction is a sudden, severe, possibly fatal allergic reaction. List five symptoms of an anaphylactic reaction.

   a. _____
   b. _____
   c. _____
   d. _____
   e. _____

24. If a UAP is working in a community setting and an individual experiences an anaphylactic reaction, the UAP must immediately make an _____ _____ _____ to the police and/or ambulance.

25. List the three medications or substances that are the most common causes of anaphylactic reaction.

    a. _____
    b. _____
    c. _____

26. An individual who has had an anaphylactic reaction to a substance should always wear a _____ to identify the substance to which he is allergic.

27. Individuals who have had a hypersensitivity reaction to a substance are at a _____ risk for reactions to other substances and require _____ _____.

28. Adverse reactions may be dangerous and even life threatening at times. The textbook lists five special considerations the UAP should follow when giving medication. List these considerations.

    a. _____
    b. _____
    c. _____
    d. _____
    e. _____

29. Medication administration among the elderly is especially challenging. Since each individual ages differently, each individual will _____ _____ to medications, including _____ to medications.

30. List the two factors the UAP must consider when administering medications to the elderly.

    a. _____
    b. _____

31. Aging is not a _____. Aging is a normal, _____ process that occurs in all individuals. Aging is _____. In other words, it begins when we are young and builds upon itself as we slowly age.

32. The UAP has the responsibility of understanding the aging process. List four things the UAP should assist the individual in his care with.

    a. _____
    b. _____
    c. _____
    d. _____

33. List the four body processes that change as an individual ages.

a. _____

b. _____

c. _____

d. _____

34. When administering medications, UAPs must be aware of their responsibility to prevent adverse reactions. This is especially true when administering medications to residents in a nursing home setting. List three special considerations for administering medications to residents living in a nursing home.

a. _____

b. _____

c. _____

MATCHING

Draw a line from each term on the left to its description in the right column.

35. inadequate absorption

36. impaired distribution

37. slower metabolism

38. impaired excretion

39. Wrong Individual

40. Wrong Medication

41. Wrong Dose

42. Wrong Time

43. Wrong Documentation

44. Wrong Route

a. the liver is less effective in filtering medications

b. the kidneys, lungs, and/or bowels are less effective at removing wastes from the body

c. the cardiovascular system works poorly so transportation of medication through the body is inadequate

d. the GI tract is slowed or the amount of fluids taken in is reduced

e. an individual was given a medication that was not prescribed for him

f. an individual was prescribed to get 50 mg of a medication and got 5 mg instead

g. nose drops were placed in the eye

h. an individual was given another individual's medication

i. medication was given at the wrong time or not at all; includes a forgotten or missed medication

j. documentation was completed incorrectly

QUESTIONS

Using what you have learned from the textbook, answer each question with one or two phrases or short sentences.

45. Is medication found on the floor a medication error? What should the UAP do about medication found on the floor?

_____

46. What should the UAP do about skipping a dose of medication? _____

_____

47. What must the UAP do if he notices that prescription medication is missing?

_____

48. What should the UAP do if he notices that OTC medication is missing?

_____

49. Is an individual's refusal to take medication considered a medication error? What should the UAP do if an individual refuses to take his medication? _____

_____

COMPLETION

Complete the following statements by filling in the blanks.

50. List four ways to prevent the misinterpretation of a licensed health care provider's order.

   a. _____

   b. _____

   c. _____

   d. _____

51. List the four steps to follow if a medication error occurs.

   a. _____

   b. _____

   c. _____

   d. _____

52. Following is a sample of a medication occurrence report (Figure 30-1), a form used when a medication error occurs. Complete the form using the following information:

   - The name of the agency is Tri-County Health Care.
   - The address of the agency is 765 Main Street, Howard, MA 01234.
   - The telephone number of the agency is (987) 654-3210.
   - The DPH registration number of the agency is 123-45-6789.

- The date and time of the occurrence are April 15, 2010, at 8 a.m.
- The name of the individual is Philip Glass.
- Philip Glass has an order for a new medication. The order reads: Penicillin VK oral suspension 250 mg oral tid × 10 days.
- Philip was supposed to get penicillin VK oral suspension 2 teaspoons at 8 a.m. This is a new medication for him. The staff member giving the medication overlooked the new medication order. Philip Glass did not get his 8 a.m. dose of penicillin VK.
- When the staff member was giving Philip his afternoon medications, the staff member realized that Philip had missed the 8 a.m. dose of penicillin VK. The staff member contacted Philip's licensed health care provider at 1:30 p.m. on April 15, 2001.
- Philip's licensed health care provider is Dr. Marcy Stone. She recommended that the staff member give Philip his next dose of penicillin VK and continue to give him the penicillin VK as ordered 3 times a day for 10 days. No medical intervention was required.

Note that the section entitled "Supervisory Review/Follow-up" is completed by your supervisor after he completes an internal investigation of the error.

53. Medication reconciliation is done every time there is a change in the individual's care; for instance, medication reconciliation is done whenever an individual is _____, _____, or _____.

54. Medication reconciliation is done to prevent medication errors caused by _____, _____, _____, or _____ _____. (Joint Commission, January 2010)

55. According to the Joint Commission, medication reconciliation consists of five steps. List the five steps.

   a. _____
   b. _____
   c. _____
   d. _____
   e. _____

56. Medication losses may create problems for the caregiver and for the individuals whose medication is missing. List two problems that may arise from a medication loss.

   a. _____
   b. _____

57. List four reasons why an individual may refuse a medication.

   a. _____
   b. _____
   c. _____
   d. _____

Department of Public Health
Medication Administration Program
MEDICATION OCCURRENCE REPORT

Agency Name:_____   Name:_____
                                                  (Consumer/Client) Last   First
Site Address:_____   Date/Time of Occurrence:_____
              Street   Site Telephone Number(____)_____
                                                 DPH Registration Number_____
_____
City/Town   Zip Code

TYPE of OCCURRENCE:
(As per regulation, contact consultant.)

(1)_____ **Wrong Individual**   (4)_____ **Wrong Dose**
(2)_____ **Wrong Medication** (includes medication given without an order)   (5)_____ **Wrong Route**
(3)_____ **Wrong Time** (includes a "forgotten "dose)

MEDICATION(S) INVOLVED:
            Name: Dosage: Frequency/Time: Route:
As Ordered:_____
As Given:_____
As Ordered:_____
As Given:_____
As Ordered:_____
As Given:_____

CONSULTANT CONTACTED
_____ Registered Nurse   _____ Registered Pharmacist   _____ Licensed Practitioner

Name of Consultant:_____ **Date Contacted:**_____ **Time Contacted:**_____
                         Last   First
Recommended Action (Medical Intervention) _____Yes _____No
If Yes, check all those that apply:
(1)_____Lab Work or Other Tests (2)_____Physician Visit (3)_____Clinic Visit (4)_____Emergency Room Visit (5)_____Hospitalization
(6)_____Other (describe)_____

Did ☐ medical intervention, ☐ illness, ☐ injury or ☐ death follow the Occurrence? ___Yes ___No

If yes, notify DPH at (617) 983-6782 /FAX(617) 524-8062 within 24 hours. For ALL Occurrences, forward written reports to your DMH/DMR MAP Coordinator within 7 days. (See reverse side for addresses.)

Supervisory Review/Follow-up
Contributing Factors: Check all that apply. If none apply, check none (g):

(a)___Failure to Accurately Record and/or Transcribe an Order   (d)___Medication Had Been Discontinued
(b)___Failure to Properly Document Administration   (e)___Improperly Labeled by Pharmacy
(c)___Medication Administered by Non-Certified Staff (Includes   (f)___Medication not Available (Explain below)
       instances where certification has expired or has been revoked)   (g)___None

_____
_____
_____(If additional space is required, please use reverse side).

Signature/Title:_____ Print Name:_____ Date:_____

0/30/96   **Occurrence Reporting is required by regulation at 105CMR 700.003(F)(1)(f).**
MAP9705.DOC   **Consultant Contact is required by regulation at 105CMR 700.003(F)(1)(g).**

DCP MAP Policy Manual May 2007

Figure 30-1 Sample Medication Error Report *(Delmar/Cengage Learning)*

58. Whatever the reason is for an individual's refusal to take a medication, _____ and _____ may help the UAP to better understand the individual's feelings.

59. Better understanding of the individual may help the UAP to explain _____ to the individual and _____.

60. Active refusal of a medication is when the individual _____ to take the medication.

61. Passive refusal requires closer monitoring because the individual initially _____ the medication but then _____ later.

62. Give two examples of an active medication refusal.
   a. _____
   b. _____

63. Give two examples of a passive refusal.
   a. _____
   b. _____

64. To refuse care, an individual must be able to _____ the consequences of her decision to refuse and must be _____ of all possible outcomes of the refusal.

65. List three questions the UAP should ask if an individual refuses a medication.
   a. _____
   b. _____
   c. _____

66. List four ways to deal with a medication refusal.
   a. _____
   b. _____
   c. _____
   d. _____

SUMMARY

Any medication may have a serious and immediate effect on an individual's health at any time. This could be caused by an allergic reaction or by a medication interaction. The UAP needs to carefully observe an individual to whom he has given medication and must report any unusual reactions right away. The UAP must also know the emergency procedures for the setting in which he works. If an emergency occurs, he must immediately follow the emergency procedures.

Chapter 31
Poison Control

Learning Objectives

After completing the following exercises, you should be able to:

1. Spell and define terms.
2. List two groups of individuals at the greatest risk for accidental poisoning.
3. List four forms poisons are found in.
4. List ten of the most dangerous poisons.
5. Explain why prevention is the best form of treatment.
6. Describe the treatment for ingestion of a poison.
7. Describe the treatment for the inhalation of a poison.
8. Describe the treatment for poisoning of the skin and eyes.
9. List thirteen steps for the emergency care of an individual with an accidental poisoning.
10. List the documentation guidelines for an accidental poisoning.
11. Describe a poison control center.

INTRODUCTION

The exercises you complete in this chapter address the following key concepts from the textbook chapter:

- forms of various poisons
- the most dangerous poisons by type and substance
- treatment for poisoning by various methods
- emergency care for an individual who has been accidentally poisoned
- documentation of an accidental poisoning
- the setup of a poison control center

VOCABULARY

Define the following terms.

1. poison _____

2. ingestion _____

3. inhalation _____

4. ocular exposure _____

5. dermal exposure _____

6. emetic _____

7. asphyxiation _____

8. vomitus _____

COMPLETION

Complete the following statements by filling in the blanks.

9. According to the American Association of Poison Control Centers, or AAPCC, _____ under the age of _____ are at the highest risk for accidental poisoning.

10. A second group at risk for poisoning is the _____.

11. If an elderly individual accidentally takes a medication overdose, this may result in _____.

12. List four reasons an elder is at risk for poisoning.

    a. _____

    b. _____

    c. _____

    d. _____

13. Poisons are found in four different forms. List the four forms.

    a. _____

    b. _____

    c. _____

    d. _____

There are five categories of poisons that the AAPCC believes are the most dangerous. Following is a list of those five categories. Read the following list. Under each category, write three examples of each type of poison.

14. Category: medicines and vitamins

    a. _____

    b. _____

    c. _____

15. Category: household products

    a. _____

    b. _____

    c. _____

16. Category: personal care products

    a. _____

    b. _____

    c. _____

17. Category: plants

    a. _____

    b. _____

    c. _____

18. Category: environmental poisons

    a. _____

    b. _____

    c. _____

QUESTIONS

Using what you have learned from the textbook, answer these questions.

19. What is the most common method of poisoning? _____

20. What is the usual treatment for an individual who has swallowed the wrong medication or too much medication? _____

21. What is the usual treatment for an individual who has swallowed a substance that is not food or medication? _____

22. Why is Ipecac no longer the drug of choice for poisoning by ingestion? _____

23. What is an individual's licensed health care provider's main concern when she is treating an individual for poisoning by inhalation? _____

24. What does the treatment for poisoning by inhalation include? _____

25. In an individual who has had an accidental poisoning by exposure to the eyes or skin, what kind(s) of treatment will be given? _____

COMPLETION

Complete the following statements by filling in the blanks.

26. Briefly describe a poison control center, including staff, availability, and what they may recommend for treatment. _____

27. List seven concerns that poison control center staff members are able to address.

   a. _____
   b. _____
   c. _____
   d. _____
   e. _____
   f. _____
   g. _____

CLINICAL SCENARIO

Read the following clinical scenario. Answer the questions that follow.

Your assignment today includes visiting Ralph, a 40-year-old man with schizophrenia who lives in supportive housing. When you arrive at his apartment, he does not answer the door. You knock and enter. There are no lights on, but you hear noise in the bathroom. When you enter the bathroom, you find Ralph on the floor. He has vomit on his shirt. His eyes are half-closed. His breathing is very slow and irregular. On the floor next to him, you see an empty bottle of cough syrup. The protective wrapping from the top is also on the floor. The label reads, "Acme Cough Suppressant—WARNING: Contains codeine." On the bathroom counter is a note from Ralph that says: "I'm through here. Sorry for the mess."

28. What is the first thing you should do? _____

29. Who should you call? _____

30. What information should you have ready when you make the phone call? _____

31. What is your next step? _____

32. You have followed the treatment instructions from the poison control center. Ralph remains unresponsive with slow, irregular breathing. Will you take Ralph to the emergency room? If so, what will you take with you? _____

33. What do you need to do last? _____

34. Write a progress note documenting this event. Use today's date and a time of 9:30 a.m. Presume, based on your observations, that Ralph has ingested the entire bottle of cough syrup. Also presume that you have already completed the incident report required by your workplace. _____

SUMMARY

Part of the UAP's responsibility is to create and maintain a safe environment for the individuals in his care. Having a good understanding of poison risks and treatment and knowing the emergency procedures before an emergency occurs will help the UAP to fulfill that responsibility to the individuals in his care.

MODULE 7
ADDITIONAL KNOWLEDGE AND SKILLS

Chapter 32
Basic Math

Learning Objectives

After completing the exercises in this chapter, you should be able to:

1. Spell and define terms.
2. Express Arabic numerals as Roman numerals.
3. Express Roman numerals as Arabic numerals.
4. Define apothecary system.
5. Define household system.
6. Define the metric system.
7. Calculate oral forms of adult medication dosages.

INTRODUCTION

The exercises you complete in this chapter will address the following key concepts from the textbook chapter:

- Arabic numerals
- Roman numerals
- apothecary system
- household system
- metric system
- oral forms of adult medication dosages

VOCABULARY

Define the following terms.

1. liter _____
2. household system _____
   _____
   _____
   _____
3. volume _____
4. Arabic numerals _____
5. meter _____
6. numerals _____
7. apothecary system _____
8. Roman numerals _____
9. gram _____
10. metric system _____

COMPLETION

Complete the following statements by filling in the blanks.

11. Medication orders are usually written in _____ numerals.
12. The health care industry uses three systems of measurement. List these three systems.
    a. _____
    b. _____
    c. _____
13. The _____ system is the old pharmacy system and is rarely used today.
14. Although the _____ system is not widely used throughout the health care industry, it is used in a home care setting or when the UAP is teaching an individual in self-administration.

15. Because the size of a drop differs from one dropper to another, it is important to use the dropper that comes with the medication. List five factors that determine the size of a drop.

   a. _____
   b. _____
   c. _____
   d. _____
   e. _____

16. The _____ system is widely used when ordering and measuring medications.

17. The basic units of the metric system are _____ for weight, _____ for volume, and _____ for length.

18. There may be times when the UAP may need to determine the amount of medication he needs to administer to an individual. List two ways the UAP can determine the amount of medication to administer.

   a. _____
   b. _____

ARABIC AND ROMAN NUMERALS

Convert the following Arabic numerals to Roman numerals.

19. 22 _____
20. 16 _____
21. 9 _____
22. 3 _____
23. 62 _____

Convert the following Roman numerals to Arabic numerals.

24. IV _____
25. XII _____
26. V _____
27. VII _____
28. XX _____

APOTHECARY AND HOUSEHOLD SYSTEMS

Write the abbreviations for each of the following:

29. gallon _____
30. drops _____
31. pint _____
32. teaspoon _____
33. ounce _____

Write in the correct abbreviation for each of the following:

34. 2 _____ = 1 oz

35. 1 _____ = 6 tsp

36. 16 _____ = 2 C

37. 4 _____ = 2 pt

38. 2 _____ = ½ gal

METRIC SYSTEM

Write in the correct equivalent for each of the following:

39. 2500 mL _____ liter

40. 3 L _____ milliliters

41. 2 g _____ mg

42. 1000 mg _____ gram

Write the correct abbreviation and unit of measurement for each of the following:

43. two grams _____

44. one thousand milligrams _____

45. two liters _____

46. 250 milliliters _____

CALCULATING ADULT ORAL DOSAGES

Calculate the correct number of tablets or capsules to be administered. Tablets are scored.

47. Order: *Urecholine 15 mg by mouth tid.*

    Available: Urecholine 10-mg tablets.

    Give: _____ tablet(s)

48. Order: *hydrochlorothiazide 12.5 mg by mouth tid.*

    Available: Hydrochlorothiazide 25-mg tablets.

    Give: _____ tablet(s)

49. Order: *Lanoxin 0.125 mg by mouth daily.*

    Available: Lanoxin 0.25-mg tablets.

    Give: _____ tablet(s)

50. Order: *Motrin 600 mg by mouth bid.*

    Available: Motrin 300-mg tablets.

    Give: _____ tablet(s)

51. Order: *Slow-K 16 mEq by mouth stat.*

    Available: Slow-K 8-mEq tablets

    Give: _____ tablet(s)

52. Order: *Cytoxan 50 mg by mouth daily.*

Available: Cytoxan 25-mg tablets.

Give: _____ tablet(s)

53. Order: *Zaroxolyn 7.5 mg by mouth bid.*

Available: Zaroxolyn 5-mg tablets.

Give: _____ tablet(s)

54. Order: *Coumadin 5 mg by mouth daily.*

Available: Coumadin 2.5-mg tablets.

Give: _____ tablet(s)

55. Order: *Trandate 150 mg by mouth bid.*

Available: Trandate 300-mg tablets

Give: _____ tablet(s)

56. Order: *Duricef 1 g by mouth bid.*

Available: Duricef 500-mg capsules

Give: _____ capsule(s)

57. Order: *Tranxene 7.5 mg by mouth qid.*

Available: Tranxene 3.75-mg capsules.

Give: _____ capsule(s)

58. Order: *Inderal 15 mg by mouth tid.*

Available: Inderal 10-mg tablets

Give: _____ tablet(s)

CALCULATING LIQUID DOSAGES

Calculate the correct amount of liquid medication to be administered.

59. Order: *Demerol syrup 75 mg by mouth q4h prn pain.*

Available: Demerol syrup 50 mg per 5 mL

Give: _____ mL

60. Order: *Pen-Vee K 1 g by mouth 1h pre-op dental surgery.*

Available: Pen-Vee K suspension 250 mg per 5 mL

Give: _____ mL

61. Order: *Tylenol 0.5 g by mouth q4h prn pain.*

Available: Tylenol 500 mg in 5 mL

Give: _____ t

62. Order: *Pathocil 125 mg by mouth q6h.*

Available: Pathocil suspension 62.5 mg per 5 mL

Give: _____ t

63. Order: *Ceclor suspension 225 mg by mouth bid.*

   Available: Ceclor suspension 375 mg per 5 mL

   Give: _____ mL

64. Order: *Septra-DS suspension 200 mg by mouth bid.*

   Available: Septra-DS suspension 400 mg per 5 mL

   Give: _____ mL

65. Order: *Trilisate liquid 750 mg by mouth tid.*

   Available: Trilisate liquid 250 mg/2.5 mL

   Give: _____ mL

66. Order: *Esidrix solution 100 mg by mouth bid.*

   Available: Esidrix solution 50 mg/5 mL

   Give: _____ t

SUMMARY

To administer medications safely and effectively, the UAP needs to have a solid foundation in the basic skills of mathematics.

Chapter 33
Vital Signs

Learning Objectives

After completing the exercises in this chapter, you should be able to:

1. Spell and define terms.
2. Identify the equipment used to take an individual's vital signs.
3. Identify the range of normal values for each type of vital sign.
4. Demonstrate measuring temperature with an oral thermometer.
5. Demonstrate measuring temperature with a rectal thermometer.
6. Demonstrate measuring temperature with a tympanic thermometer.
7. Demonstrate counting a radial pulse.
8. Demonstrate counting an apical pulse.
9. Demonstrate counting respirations.
10. Demonstrate taking blood pressure using a standard blood pressure cuff and stethoscope.
11. Demonstrate taking a blood pressure with an automatic blood pressure unit.

INTRODUCTION

The exercises you complete in this chapter will address the following key concepts from the textbook chapter:

- the equipment used to take blood pressure, temperature, pulse, and respirations
- measuring temperature with various types of thermometers
- counting pulse and respirations
- measuring blood pressure with various types of equipment

VOCABULARY

Define the following terms.

1. vital signs _____
2. temperature _____
3. body core _____
4. oral temperature _____
5. tympanic temperature _____
6. rectal temperature _____
7. axillary temperature _____
8. probe _____
9. pulse _____
10. radial pulse _____
11. apical pulse _____
12. pedal pulse _____
13. respiration _____
14. systolic blood pressure _____
15. diastolic blood pressure _____

COMPLETION

Complete the following statements by filling in the blanks.

16. After taking an individual's vital signs, the UAP should complete three steps. List the three steps the UAP should complete.

    a. _____
    b. _____
    c. _____

17. An individual's body temperature may be affected by many different factors. List five of those factors.

a. _____
b. _____
c. _____
d. _____
e. _____

18. Temperatures are typically measured orally. However, there are times when taking an oral temperature is not safe or accurate. List six circumstances when a UAP should *not* use an oral thermometer.

a. _____
b. _____
c. _____
d. _____
e. _____
f. _____

19. There are times when a licensed health care provider orders a temperature to be taken by a different route, such as a rectal temperature. However, there are times when taking a rectal temperature is not safe or accurate. List four circumstances when a UAP should *not* use a rectal thermometer.

a. _____
b. _____
c. _____
d. _____

MATCHING

Draw lines to connect each term in the left column with its definition in the right column.

20. tympanic thermometer

21. disposable oral thermometer

22. digital thermometer

23. electronic thermometer

a. reads a temperature in about 30 seconds

b. reads a temperature in 20 to 60 seconds

c. reads a temperature in just a few seconds

d. could cause tears in the lips and mouth if taken out while the mouth is closed

COMPLETION

Complete the following statements by filling in the blanks.

24. The pulse is the pressure of the blood against an artery wall as the heart beats. There are four common areas for taking a pulse. List each area. Include the specific name of the pulse measured at each area.

    a. _____
    b. _____
    c. _____
    d. _____

25. There are two characteristics used to describe an individual's pulse. They are the _____ and _____ of the pulse.

26. The term "bradycardia" describes a pulse rate that is _____
    _____.

27. The term "tachycardia" describes a pulse rate that is _____
    _____
    _____.

28. When describing an individual's pulse, it is important to note irregularities in character. Define the character of a pulse. _____
    _____

29. The volume of a pulse is the fullness of the beat. Give two descriptions of a pulse volume.

    a. _____
    b. _____

30. Pulse rates may be affected by many different factors. List six factors that may make a pulse rate higher or lower.

    a. _____
    b. _____
    c. _____
    d. _____
    e. _____
    f. _____

MATCHING

Draw lines to connect each term in the left column with its definition in the right column.

31. inspiration
32. expiration
33. rate
34. rhythm
35. symmetry
36. volume
37. normal breathing
38. tachypnea
39. shallow
40. dyspnea
41. apnea
42. Cheyne-Stokes
43. stertorous
44. rales
45. wheezing

a. whether the chest expands equally on both sides as air enters the lungs
b. number of respirations per minute
c. depth of the respiration
d. breathing in
e. regularity of breathing
f. breathing out
g. a breath that only partially fills the lungs
h. a repeating pattern of dyspnea and apnea
i. respirations that are similar to snoring
j. a moist respiration caused by fluid in the air passages
k. 16 to 20 breaths per minute
l. dyspnea with a sighing or whistling sound
m. a period of no respirations
n. fast, shallow breathing
o. difficult or labored breathing

COMPLETION

Complete the following statements by filling in the blanks.

46. Blood pressure measures the force of the blood against the walls of the arteries during a heartbeat. There are many factors that may affect an individual's blood pressure from day to day. List six factors that may make a blood pressure higher.

   a. _____
   b. _____
   c. _____
   d. _____
   e. _____
   f. _____

47. List five factors that may make a blood pressure lower.

   a. _____
   b. _____
   c. _____
   d. _____
   e. _____

48. Because each individual is different, their habits and lifestyles affect their blood pressures. List five factors that may affect an individual's typical blood pressure reading.

a. _____
b. _____
c. _____
d. _____
e. _____

49. There are many causes of an inaccurate blood pressure reading. List four causes for an inaccurate reading.

a. _____
b. _____
c. _____
d. _____

CHOICES

50. From the list below, circle the pieces of equipment needed to take an individual's oral or rectal temperature.

thermometer	stethoscope	clean paper tissue
watch with a second hand	disposable probe covers	paper or notepad
gloves	alcohol wipes	sphygmomanometer
pen	lubricant	

51. From the list below, circle the pieces of equipment needed to take an individual's pulse and respirations.

clean paper tissue	watch with a second hand	disposable probe covers
stethoscope	paper or notepad	thermometer
alcohol wipes	gloves	pen

52. From the list below, circle the pieces of equipment needed to take an individual's blood pressure.

watch with a second hand	disposable probe covers	clean paper tissue
sphygmomanometer	gloves	thermometer
pen	stethoscope	alcohol wipes
paper or notepad	lubricant	

PRACTICAL APPLICATIONS

53. Write the names of the thermometers pictured.

   a. _____

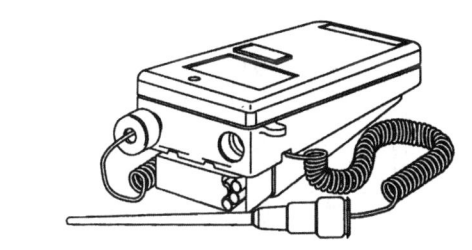

   b. _____

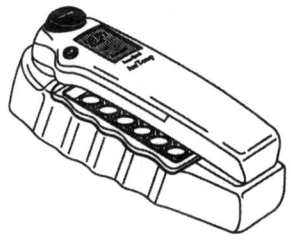

54. Determine the systolic and diastolic readings.

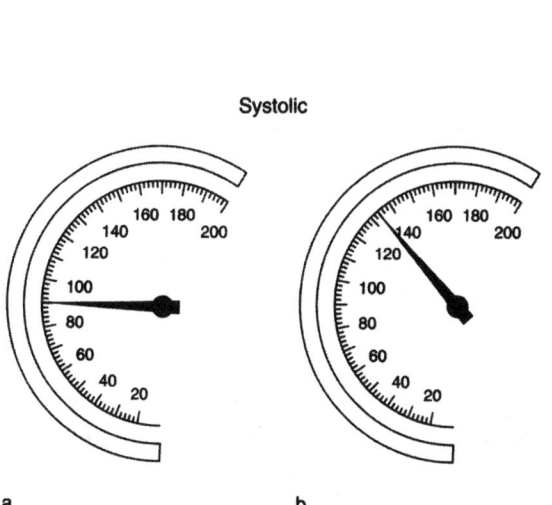

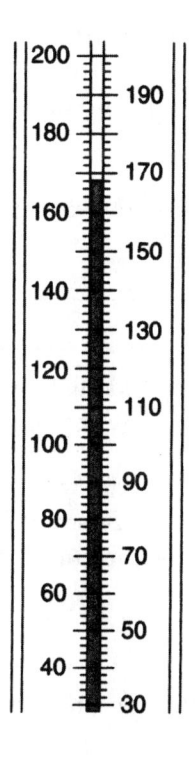

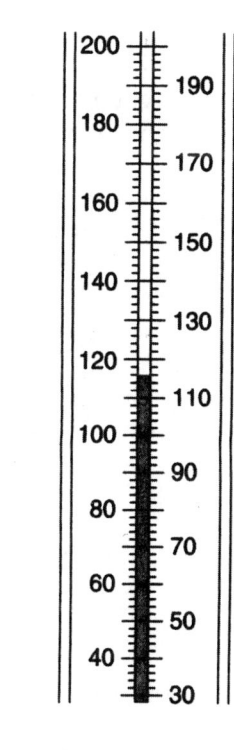

a. _____ b. _____ c. _____ d. _____

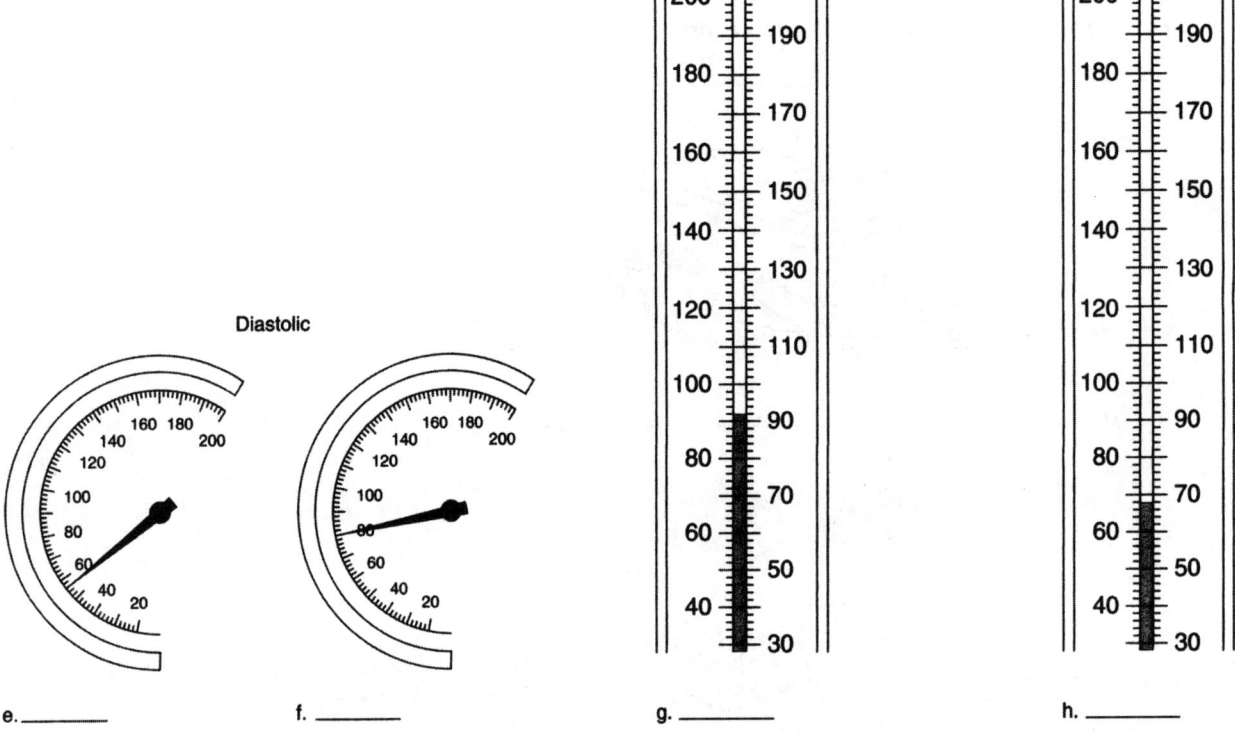

e. _____ f. _____ g. _____ h. _____

You are asked to take Mr. Harrison's vital signs as part of your assignment. Mr. Harrison is a new individual at your workplace. He is at your workplace for a short-term respite stay. When you are gathering information about him, you see that he has a diagnosis of Alzheimer's disease. When you approach him to introduce yourself, you see that he is fidgeting and restless. When you say, "Hello, Mr. Harrison," he says, "I'm just here to catch the bus home. I'm just here to catch the bus."

55. Do you think that it would be a good idea to take Mr. Harrison's temperature orally? If so, why? If not, why not?

_____

_____

56. When you check his licensed HCP orders, you do not see any orders for taking a temperature other than orally. What do you do now? _____

_____

57. After speaking to your supervisor, it is determined that a tympanic temperature reading would be safe. Why would this be better than taking an oral temperature?

_____

_____

58. Describe how you would measure Mr. Harrison's temperature with a tympanic thermometer. _____

_____

_____

59. Now you are going to count Mr. Harrison's pulse and respirations. Do you think these readings are going to be high, low, or average? Why? _____
_____
_____

60. Describe the steps you would take to count Mr. Harrison's pulse and respirations. ___
_____
_____
_____
_____

61. Now you are going to measure Mr. Harrison's blood pressure. Do you think this will be high, low, or average? Why?
_____
_____

62. What steps should you take to prepare before measuring Mr. Harrison's blood pressure? _____
_____
_____
_____

63. When you are writing down Mr. Harrison's blood pressure, what information should you include? Why? _____
_____
_____
_____

SUMMARY

Taking vital signs is an important way of quickly gathering information about an individual. A change in an individual's vital signs may signal an oncoming illness or medical issue. Taking vital signs is one of the many skills the UAP may use to communicate effectively with her supervisor and the licensed HCP about the individuals in her care.

Chapter 34
Care of Individuals with Epilepsy

Learning Objectives

After completing the following exercises, you should be able to:

1. Spell and define terms.
2. Briefly describe the changes that occur in the body because of epilepsy.
3. List five possible causes of epilepsy.
4. Describe two major categories of seizures.
5. Describe emergency care of an individual having a seizure.
6. Explain why status epilepticus is a medical emergency.
7. Demonstrate the administration of Diastat gel.
8. Briefly describe four methods of treatment for an individual who has epilepsy.
9. List six anticonvulsants, their routes, side effects, and special considerations.
10. Explain the danger of discontinuing anticonvulsant medication for an individual who is in remission.
11. Describe a VNS implant and how it works.

INTRODUCTION

The exercises you complete in this chapter address the following key concepts from the textbook chapter:

- causes of epilepsy and the changes that occur in the body as a result of epilepsy
- various types of seizures that may be experienced by an individual with epilepsy
- emergency care for an individual who is having an epileptic seizure
- the emergency nature of status epilepticus
- administration of Diastat gel
- medications used to treat epilepsy, including side effects and consequences of discontinuation
- other treatments for epilepsy, including surgery, ketogenic diet, use of a VNS implant, and complementary treatments
- care of the individual with epilepsy

VOCABULARY

Define the following terms.

1. epilepsy _____

2. seizures _____

3. anticonvulsant medications _____

4. therapeutic range _____

5. remission _____

COMPLETION

Complete the following statements by filling in the blanks.

6. Epilepsy affects individuals of all ages, races, and ethnic backgrounds. Epilepsy is not a mental disorder. Epilepsy is a disorder of the _____ system.

7. Epilepsy is a _____ disorder caused by _____ _____ _____ and _____ periods of _____ brain activity.

8. Epilepsy is treatable with _____, _____, _____, and/or a device that _____ the _____ nerve.

9. Once under treatment, epilepsy does not _____ with age.

10. Epilepsy causes a disruption in the electrical charges in the brain. This disruption may cause physical changes in an individual for a short period of time. These physical changes are called _____.

11. List three effects seizures may have on the body.

    a. _____
    b. _____
    c. _____

12. A single seizure does not mean that an individual has epilepsy. It is only when the seizures _____ or when the problem causing the seizures cannot be _____ that the seizure disorder is called epilepsy.

13. List five possible causes of epilepsy.

    a. _____
    b. _____
    c. _____
    d. _____
    e. _____

14. Seizures are physical changes in the body due to disruption of electrical charges in the brain. Depending on the area of the brain where the disruption occurs, seizures will look different. List three physical changes a UAP may see when an individual has a seizure.

    a. _____
    b. _____
    c. _____

15. The goal of seizure treatment is always to _____ the seizures with the least amount of _____ possible.

16. An aura may occur in some individuals just before they _____.

17. An aura involves an individual's _____.

18. When an aura occurs, the UAP caring for the individual should _____.

QUESTIONS

Using what you have learned from the textbook, answer these questions.

19. What is the difference between partial and generalized seizures? _____
_____
_____

20. Considering partial and generalized seizures, which is the more common type of seizure? _____

21. Which is the most common type of generalized seizure? _____
_____

22. What are four main types of generalized seizures?
    a. _____
    b. _____
    c. _____
    d. _____

23. What are three facts to remember about partial seizures?
    a. _____
    b. _____
    c. _____

24. What are three facts to remember about generalized tonic-clonic seizures?
    a. _____
    b. _____
    c. _____

MATCHING

There are many different types of seizures. Although each type of seizure has the same basic characteristics, seizures look different from one individual to the next.

Draw lines to connect each term in the left column with its definition in the right column.

25. partial seizure
26. generalized seizure
27. nonepileptic seizure
28. myoclonic seizure
29. atonic seizure
30. absence seizure

a. caused by a physical condition, emotional trauma, or psychological stress; not related to epilepsy

b. a seizure in which there is a sudden loss of muscle tone; also called a "drop attack"

c. a seizure in which an individual experiences a lapse in awareness

d. limited to one side of the brain; an individual may or may not lose consciousness

e. affects both sides of the brain from the beginning of the seizure

f. a seizure consisting of rapid, brief muscle contractions that occur at the same time on both sides of the body

CLINICAL SCENARIOS

Read the following clinical scenarios. Answer the questions.

Part of your assignment today is to give care to Ron. Ron has had epilepsy for the last seven years. Ron is having breakfast and talking to you. He suddenly stops talking in midsentence. When you look at him, you see that he is staring off into space. Ron begins to mumble and pick at his clothing. You ask what he is doing. He replies, "I'm picking nits, picking nits, picking nits." You step toward Ron to assist him. He sees you coming and jumps up from his chair. Ron stands beside the table, flapping his hands and saying, "picking nits, picking nits, picking nits."

31. What is happening to Ron? _____

32. Explain what you would do to keep Ron safe during this event. _____

You are working in a group home. Joan is one of the residents. She has had epilepsy for the last three years. Joan is in the bathroom, getting ready to leave for an outing. You hear a loud thud from the bathroom. When you knock on the door, Joan does not answer. You go in and find Joan lying on the floor. Her arms, legs, and trunk are all stiff. As you approach her, Joan's legs begin to jerk.

33. What is happening to Joan? _____

34. Should you help Joan to get up and move to her bedroom? Why or why not? If not, explain how Joan should be positioned during this event. _____

35. Explain what you would do to keep Joan safe during this event. _____

QUESTIONS

Using what you have learned from the textbook, answer these questions.

36. What is status epilepticus? _____

37. Why is status epilepticus an emergency? _____

38. What three actions should the UAP take when caring for an individual with epilepsy, especially when caring for an individual with a history of status epilepticus?

    a. _____
    b. _____
    c. _____

39. What is the treatment of choice for status epilepticus? _____

40. What is the first choice of treatment for epilepsy? _____

COMPLETION

Complete the following statements by filling in the blanks.

41. List six classes of medications that are used to treat epilepsy. Briefly describe the type(s) of seizures each class of medication treats.

    a. _____
    b. _____
    c. _____
    d. _____
    e. _____
    f. _____

42. List four of the *most common* side effects of anticonvulsant medications.

    a. _____
    b. _____
    c. _____
    d. _____

43. List six of the warning signs of *possible serious* side effects of anticonvulsant medications.

   a. _____
   b. _____
   c. _____
   d. _____
   e. _____
   f. _____

44. A serious concern with anticonvulsant medications is the difference between brand-name medications and generic medications. Briefly describe the differences between a brand-name and generic medication that causes this concern.

   _____
   _____
   _____
   _____

45. List the four criteria for surgery in treating an individual with epilepsy.

   a. _____
   b. _____
   c. _____
   d. _____

46. Briefly explain how a ketogenic diet works for an individual with epilepsy.

   _____
   _____
   _____
   _____

47. Briefly explain how VNS therapy works for an individual with epilepsy.

   _____
   _____
   _____
   _____

48. List five side effects that an individual with a VNS implant may have.

   a. _____
   b. _____
   c. _____
   d. _____
   e. _____

49. List two forms of complementary or alternative treatments for an individual with epilepsy.

   a. _____

   b. _____

50. List four responsibilities the UAP has when caring for an individual with epilepsy.

   a. _____

   b. _____

   c. _____

   d. _____

51. Briefly describe how to give mouth care to an individual who is on long-term Dilantin therapy. _____

SUMMARY

Giving care to an individual with epilepsy may appear to be an overwhelming task for the UAP. Providing emergency care during a seizure, administering medications to control seizures, and monitoring the individual for any changes related to medications or seizure activity are the responsibility of the UAP in his role as caregiver. If the UAP has a good understanding of these tasks, as well as a strong foundation of clinical skills, he should be able to perform his tasks smoothly and give the best care possible.

Chapter 35
Substance Abuse

Learning Objectives

After completing the exercises in this chapter, you should be able to:

1. Spell and define key terms.
2. Describe four commonly abused substances in the United States today.
3. List three routes of administration for abused substances.
4. List the street names for six commonly abused substances in the United States.
5. Describe five adverse reactions due to the use of abused substances.
6. Discuss the role of the UAP in recognizing and reporting suspected substance abuse.

INTRODUCTION

The exercises you complete in this chapter will address the following key concepts from the textbook chapter:

- commonly abused substances
- routes of administration for abused substances
- street names for six commonly abused substances
- adverse reactions due to the use of abused substances
- responsibilities of the UAP regarding suspected substance abuse

VOCABULARY

1. psychotropic _____
2. substance abuse _____
3. addiction _____
4. physical addiction _____
5. psychological addiction _____
6. withdrawal _____
7. anterograde amnesia _____
8. huffing _____

COMPLETION

Complete the following statements by filling in the blanks.

9. Cannabinoids include _____ and _____.
10. List four symptoms of marijuana use that the UAP could observe in everyday situations.
    a. _____
    b. _____
    c. _____
    d. _____
11. List three street names for marijuana.
    a. _____
    b. _____
    c. _____
12. Depressants include both _____ _____ and _____ _____.
13. Club drugs are dangerous substances that are commonly used by _____ and _____ at parties, bars, and clubs.
14. Hallucinogens include _____ and _____.

15. Individuals who abuse LSD often experience flashbacks. Flashbacks occur _____ and without _____.

16. List four symptoms of PCP use that the UAP could observe in everyday situations.

    a. _____
    b. _____
    c. _____
    d. _____

17. Opiates that have medical uses are Schedules _____ controlled substances.

18. List three examples of opiates that have a medical use.

    a. _____
    b. _____
    c. _____

19. Stimulants include _____ _____, _____ _____, and legal substances, such as _____.

20. Cocaine is a _____.

21. List four street names for cocaine.

    a. _____
    b. _____
    c. _____
    d. _____

22. List four responses in the body that are caused by amphetamines.

    a. _____
    b. _____
    c. _____
    d. _____

23. List three street names for amphetamines.

    a. _____
    b. _____
    c. _____

24. Nicotine is highly addictive, causing withdrawal if stopped suddenly. In addition, nicotine increases an individual's risk for numerous illnesses. List four of these illnesses.

    a. _____
    b. _____
    c. _____
    d. _____

25. Anabolic steroids are man-made substances that can lead to _____, _____ health problems.

26. Dextromethorphan (DXM) is a substance found in _____ and ____ medications.

27. List four responses in the body that are caused by Dextromethorphan (DXM).

    a. _____
    b. _____
    c. _____
    d. _____

28. Inhalants are household substances that are breathed in through the _____ or _____.

29. List three household substances that may be abused as inhalants.

    a. _____
    b. _____
    c. _____

QUESTIONS

Using what you have learned from the textbook, answer each question with one or two phrases or short sentences.

30. What actions do barbiturates have in the body?

    a. _____
    b. _____

31. How is cocaine taken into the body? _____

32. What is the difference between cocaine and crack cocaine?

    _____
    _____

33. How does a psychedelic drug affect the body?_____
    _____

34. How is marijuana or hashish taken into the body? _____
    _____

35. What is the number one drug problem in the United States? _____

36. Prolonged alcohol use affects all organs of the body and can cause permanent damage. What types of damage can alcohol cause to the body?

    a. _____
    b. _____
    c. _____
    d. _____

37. What does the UAP do if he meets an individual who he thinks might be abusing substances? _____

_____

38. What if that individual is an individual to whom the UAP gives care?

_____

39. What if that individual is the UAP's coworker?_____

_____

SUMMARY

The UAP is responsible for reporting suspected substance abuse whether it is done by an individual in the UAP's care or by a coworker. Substance abuse is a serious issue of legality and safety.

SECTION 2
Performance Record and Skill Checklists

PERFORMANCE RECORD

Your instructor will observe and evaluate your performance with each procedure that you learn. The instructor will keep a record of your progress; however, you may find it helpful to keep a personal record.

PROCEDURE		DATE	SATISFACTORY	UNSATISFACTORY
Documentation Procedures				
Procedure 6-1	Handwashing			
Procedure (Optional)	Removing Gloves			
Procedure 7-1	Administration of Oral Medications			
Procedure 7-2	Administration of Ophthalmic (Eye) Medications			
Procedure 7-3	Administration of Otic (Ear) Medications			
Procedure 7-4	Administration of Nasal Medications			
Procedure 7-5	Administration of Medications for Skin and Hair			
Procedure 7-6	Administration of Transdermal Medications			
Procedure 7-7	Administration of Rectal Medications			
Procedure 7-8	Administration of Vaginal Medications			
Procedure 7-9	Administration of Medications by Inhaler			
Procedure (Optional)	Use of a Small-Volume Nebulizer			
Procedure 8-1	Use of a Pulse Oximeter			
Procedure 8-2	Changing a Humidifier Bottle			
Procedure 8-3	Use of an Incentive Spirometer			
Procedure 9-1	Administration of a Cleansing Enema			
Procedure 9-2	Administration of a Ready-to-Use (Prepackaged) Enema			
Procedure 10-1	Administration of a Continuous Tube Feeding			
Procedure 10-2	Administration of an Intermittent Feeding by Bolus			

(Continued)

SKILL CHECKLIST

Procedure 7-1 Administration of Oral Medications

Objective: To safely and effectively administer a solid and a liquid oral medication.

Instructions to the Learner: Following the licensed health care provider orders transcribed onto the medication sheet, correctly administer the oral medications as stated by your instructor.

Directions to the Instructor: Write an S or U to indicate a satisfactory or unsatisfactory performance.

PROCEDURAL STEPS	S OR U	COMMENTS
1. Identifies the right individual.		
2. Washes hands.		
3. Gathers appropriate equipment.		
4. Works in a well-lighted, quiet, clean area.		
5. Compares the medication sheet with the licensed HCP orders.		
6. Identifies the right medication and removes the medication from the storage area.		
7. Checks the expiration date.		
8. Compares the pharmacy label to the medication sheet.		
9. Prepares the right dose (a, b, and/or c): a. multiple dose solid medication b. unit dose medication c. liquid medication		
10. Calculates the dose, if necessary.		
11. Signs the count page in the Controlled Substance Count Book, if needed.		
12. Compares the pharmacy label to the medication sheet for the second time.		
13. Double-checks the medication sheet to make sure the medication is being given to the right individual.		
14. Properly carries the medication to the individual.		
15. Takes and records vital signs, if needed.		
16. Assists the individual into a comfortable position. Explains the procedure to the individual.		
17. Administers the medication by the right route. Makes sure the individual takes the medication.		
18. Provides for the individual's safety. Returns the individual to a comfortable position.		
19. Cares for equipment and supplies.		
20. Washes hands.		
21. Documents administration of the medication correctly. Compares the pharmacy label to the medication sheet a third time.		
22. Observes the individual for any unpleasant or harmful effects from the medication.		
23. Keeps medication storage areas locked at appropriate times and does not leave the areas unlocked when unattended.		

PROCEDURE		DATE	SATISFACTORY	UNSATISFACTORY
Procedure 10-3	Administration of an Intermittent Feeding by Gravity Drip Method			
Procedure 10-4	Care of Gastrostomy and Jejunostomy Tubes			
Procedure 10-5	Flushing Gastrostomy and Jejunostomy Tubes			
Procedure 10-6	Checking for Residual Feeding			
Procedure 10-7	Administration of Medication through a Gastrostomy or Jejunostomy Tube with a Continuous Feeding			
Procedure 10-8	Administration of Medication through a Gastrostomy or Jejunostomy Tube with an Intermittent Feeding			
Procedure 11-1	Administration of an EpiPen Auto-Injector			
Procedure 33-1	Taking an Oral Temperature with an Electronic or Digital Thermometer			
Procedure 33-2	Taking a Rectal Temperature with an Electronic or Digital Thermometer			
Procedure 33-3	Taking an Axillary Temperature with an Electronic or Digital Thermometer			
Procedure 33-4	Taking a Temperature with a Tympanic Thermometer			
Procedure 33-5	Counting a Radial Pulse			
Procedure (Optional)	Counting an Apical Pulse			
Procedure 33-6	Counting Respirations			
Procedure 33-7	Measuring Blood Pressure with a Sphygmomanometer and Stethoscope			
Procedure 33-8	Measuring Blood Pressure with an Electronic or an Automatic Blood Pressure Unit			
Procedure 34-1	Administration of Diastat (Diazepam)			

SKILL CHECKLIST

Documentation Procedures

Objective: To correctly complete various forms of documentation required in medication administration.

Instructions to the Learner: Following the principles and guidelines discussed in Chapters 5, 6, 29 and 30 of the textbook, perform all tasks required to successfully complete the documentation below.

Directions to the Instructor: Write an S or U to indicate a satisfactory or unsatisfactory performance.

PROCEDURAL STEPS	S OR U	COMMENTS
1. Completes a telephone order.		
2. Completes a Controlled Substance Count:		
a. Index Page		
b. Count Page		
c. Count Verification Page		
3. Completes a medication disposal form appropriate for the workplace.		
4. Completes a medication error report form appropriate for the workplace.		
5. Completes a drug incident report form appropriate for the workplace.		
6. Transcribes licensed HCP's orders onto a medication sheet:		
a. liquid medication		
b. solid medication		
7. Writes a progress note.		
8. Discontinues a medication on a medication sheet.		
9. Posts and verifies transcribed orders.		
10. Completes a monthly quality review.		

SKILL CHECKLIST

Procedure 6-1 Handwashing

Objective: To correctly perform the task of handwashing.

Instructions to the Learner: Following the principles taught in Chapter 6 of the textbook, demonstrate the task of handwashing.

Directions to the Instructor: Write an S or U to indicate a satisfactory or unsatisfactory performance.

PROCEDURAL STEPS	S OR U	COMMENTS
1. Gathers appropriate equipment: soap, paper towels, trash basket, and, if needed, an orange stick.		
2. Removes rings, if possible.		
3. Removes watch or pushes watch up over wrist. Also moves sleeves up over wrist.		
4. Turns on faucet with a dry paper towel. Adjusts water temperature. Stands so that clothing does not touch the sink.		
5. Wets hands. Keeps fingertips pointed downward at all times so water runs off fingertips.		
6. Applies adequate amount of soap (about 1 teaspoon) to hands.		
7. Lathers soap over hands and wrists, between fingers and under rings. Interlaces fingers. Works lather over every part of hands and wrists. Cleans fingernails by rubbing them against the palm of the opposite hand to force soap under the nails. Washes hands for 15 to 20 seconds.		
8. Uses an orange stick to clean under fingernails, if needed.		
9. Rinses hands well with fingertips pointed downward so water runs off fingertips. Does not shake water from hands.		
10. Dries hands and wrists thoroughly with clean paper towels. Discards each paper towel into the trash as it is used.		
11. Turns off the faucets with a clean, dry paper towel. Discards the paper towel into the trash.		
12. If needed, applies lotion to hands.		

SKILL CHECKLIST

Procedure (Optional) Removing Gloves

Objective: To correctly remove gloves.

Instructions to the Learner: Following the principles discussed in Chapter 6 of the textbook, demonstrate the task of removing gloves.

Directions to the Instructor: Write an S or U to indicate a satisfactory or unsatisfactory performance.

PROCEDURAL STEPS	S OR U	COMMENTS
1. Slips gloved fingers of one hand under the cuff of the opposite hand, touching the glove only. If the glove does not have a cuff, grabs the outer part of the glove at the wrist with the opposite gloved hand.		
2. Pulls the glove down to the fingers, uncovering the thumb.		
3. Slips the uncovered thumb under the opposite (second) glove at the wrist.		
4. Allows the glove-covered fingers of the hand to touch only the outer part of the soiled glove.		
5. Pulls the glove down over the first hand almost to the fingertips and slips the glove onto the second hand.		
6. With the first hand touching only the outside of the second hand, continues pulling the glove over the first hand until only the clean part of the glove is showing.		
7. Disposes of the soiled gloves according to work site policy.		
8. Washes and dries hands thoroughly.		

SKILL CHECKLIST

Procedure 7-2 Administration of Ophthalmic (Eye) Medications

Objective: To safely and effectively administer eyedrops and eye ointment.

Instructions to the Learner: Following the licensed health care provider orders transcribed onto the medication sheet, correctly administer the ophthalmic medications as stated by your instructor.

Directions to the Instructor: Write an S or U to indicate a satisfactory or unsatisfactory performance.

PROCEDURAL STEPS	S OR U	COMMENTS
1. Identifies the right individual.		
2. Washes hands.		
3. Gathers appropriate equipment.		
4. Works in a well-lighted, quiet, clean area.		
5. Compares the medication sheet with the licensed HCP orders.		
6. Identifies the right medication and removes the medication from the storage area.		
7. Checks the expiration date.		
8. Compares the pharmacy label to the medication sheet.		
9. Prepares the right dose (a and/or b): a. eyedrops b. eye ointment		
10. Compares the pharmacy label to the medication sheet for the second time.		
11. Double-checks the medication sheet to make sure the medication is being given to the right individual.		
12. Properly carries the medication and equipment to the individual.		
13. Assists the individual into a comfortable position.		
14. Puts on gloves. Wipes the eye and eyelid.		
15. Gently makes a "pocket" with the individual's lower eyelid.		
16. Administers the medication by the right route. Applies gentle pressure against the inner corner (nose side) of the eye.		
17. Provides for the individual's safety. Returns the individual to a comfortable position.		
18. Cares for equipment and supplies.		
19. Removes gloves. Washes hands.		
20. If administering ointment, informs the individual that his vision may be blurry from the medication.		
21. Documents administration of the medication correctly. Compares the pharmacy label to the medication sheet a third time.		
22. Observes the individual for any unpleasant or harmful effects from the medication.		
23. Keeps medication storage areas locked at appropriate times and does not leave the areas unlocked when unattended.		

SKILL CHECKLIST

Procedure 7-3 Administration of Otic (Ear) Medications

Objective: To safely and effectively administer eardrops.

Instructions to the Learner: Following the licensed health care provider orders transcribed onto the medication sheet, correctly administer the otic medication as stated by your instructor.

Directions to the Instructor: Write an S or U to indicate a satisfactory or unsatisfactory performance.

PROCEDURAL STEPS	S OR U	COMMENTS
1. Identifies the right individual.		
2. Washes hands.		
3. Gathers appropriate equipment.		
4. Works in a well-lighted, quiet, clean area.		
5. Compares the medication sheet with the licensed HCP orders.		
6. Identifies the right medication and removes the medication from the storage area.		
7. Checks the expiration date.		
8. Compares the pharmacy label to the medication sheet.		
9. Prepares the right dose. Ensures that the medication is at room temperature.		
10. Compares the pharmacy label to the medication sheet for the second time.		
11. Double-checks the medication sheet to make sure the medication is being given to the right individual.		
12. Properly carries the medication and equipment to the individual.		
13. Assists the individual into a comfortable position.		
14. Puts on gloves. Wipes the outer ear, if needed.		
15. Gently pulls the earlobe up and outward.		
16. Administers the medication by the right route. Drops the medication onto the outer part of the ear canal and lets it gently roll into the ear canal.		
17. Has the individual stay in position for 5 minutes.		
18. If licensed HCP orders, places cottonball into the individual's ear.		
19. Provides for the individual's safety. Returns the individual to a comfortable position.		
20. Cares for equipment and supplies.		
21. Removes gloves. Washes hands.		
22. Documents administration of the medication correctly. Compares the pharmacy label to the medication sheet a third time.		
23. Observes the individual for any unpleasant or harmful effects from the medication.		
24. Keeps medication storage areas locked at appropriate times and does not leave the areas unlocked when unattended.		

SKILL CHECKLIST

Procedure 7-4 Administration of Nasal Medications

Objective: To safely and effectively administer nose drops, a nasal spray, and a nasal inhaler.

Instructions to the Learner: Following the licensed health care provider orders transcribed onto the medication sheet, correctly administer the nasal medications as stated by your instructor.

Directions to the Instructor: Write an S or U to indicate a satisfactory or unsatisfactory performance.

PROCEDURAL STEPS	S OR U	COMMENTS
1. Identifies the right individual.		
2. Washes hands.		
3. Gathers appropriate equipment.		
4. Works in a well-lighted, quiet, clean area.		
5. Compares the medication sheet with the licensed HCP orders.		
6. Identifies the right medication and removes the medication from the storage area.		
7. Checks the expiration date.		
8. Compares the pharmacy label to the medication sheet.		
9. Prepares the right dose (a, b, and/or c): a. nose drops b. nasal spray c. nasal inhaler		
10. Compares the pharmacy label to the medication sheet for the second time.		
11. Double-checks the medication sheet to make sure the medication is being given to the right individual.		
12. Properly carries the medication and equipment to the individual.		
13. Assists the individual into a comfortable position.		
14. Puts on gloves. Wipes the nose, if needed.		
15. Administers the medication by the right route.		
16. Has the individual stay in position for 3 to 5 minutes.		
17. Provides for the individual's safety. Returns the individual to a comfortable position.		
18. Cares for equipment and supplies.		
19. Removes gloves. Washes hands.		
20. Documents administration of the medication correctly. Compares the pharmacy label to the medication sheet a third time.		
21. Observes the individual for any unpleasant or harmful effects from the medication.		
22. Keeps medication storage areas locked at appropriate times and does not leave the areas unlocked when unattended.		

SKILL CHECKLIST

Procedure 7-5 Administration of Medications for Skin and Hair

Objective: To safely and effectively administer topical medications to the skin and hair, including powders, lotions, tinctures, solutions, suspensions, ointments, creams, and shampoos.

Instructions to the Learner: Following the licensed health care provider orders transcribed onto the medication sheet, correctly administer the topical medications as stated by your instructor.

Directions to the Instructor: Write an S or U to indicate a satisfactory or unsatisfactory performance.

PROCEDURAL STEPS	S OR U	COMMENTS
1. Identifies the right individual.		
2. Washes hands.		
3. Gathers appropriate equipment.		
4. Works in a well-lighted, quiet, clean area.		
5. Compares the medication sheet with the licensed HCP orders.		
6. Identifies the right medication and removes the medication from the storage area.		
7. Checks the expiration date		
8. Compares the pharmacy label to the medication sheet.		
9. Prepares the right dose (a, b, c, and/or d): a. powders b. lotions, tinctures, solutions, suspensions c. creams and ointments d. shampoos		
10. Compares the pharmacy label to the medication sheet for the second time.		
11. Double-checks the medication sheet to make sure the medication is being given to the right individual.		
12. Properly carries the medication and equipment to the individual.		
13. Assists the individual into a comfortable position.		
14. Puts on gloves.		
15. Unless otherwise ordered by the licensed HCP, cleanses the area to be treated with mild soap and warm water. Rinses the area well and then gently pats the area dry with a clean cloth.		
16. If applying a medicated shampoo, first washes the individual's hair with a nonmedicated shampoo, if required.		
17. Administers the medication by the right route.		
18. Provides for the individual's safety. Returns the individual to a comfortable position.		
19. Cares for equipment and supplies.		
20. Removes gloves. Washes hands.		
21. Documents administration of the medication correctly. Compares the pharmacy label to the medication sheet a third time.		
22. Observes the individual for any unpleasant or harmful effects from the medication.		
23. Keeps medication storage areas locked at appropriate times and does not leave the areas unlocked when unattended.		

SKILL CHECKLIST

Procedure 7-6 Administration of Transdermal Medications

Objective: To safely and effectively administer transdermal medications.

Instructions to the Learner: Following the licensed health care provider orders transcribed onto the medication sheet, correctly administer the transdermal medications as stated by your instructor.

Directions to the Instructor: Write an S or U to indicate a satisfactory or unsatisfactory performance.

PROCEDURAL STEPS	S OR U	COMMENTS
1. Identifies the right individual.		
2. Washes hands.		
3. Gathers appropriate equipment.		
4. Works in a well-lighted, quiet, clean area.		
5. Compares the medication sheet with the licensed HCP orders.		
6. Identifies the right medication and removes the medication from the storage area.		
7. Checks the expiration date.		
8. Compares the pharmacy label to the medication sheet.		
9. Prepares the right dose.		
10. Compares the pharmacy label to the medication sheet for the second time.		
11. Double-checks the medication sheet to make sure the medication is being given to the right individual.		
12. Properly carries the medication and equipment to the individual.		
13. Assists the individual into a comfortable position.		
14. Puts on gloves.		
15. Administers the medication by the right route. Applies the new patch to a new area of the body. Dates and initials the new patch.		
16. Removes the old patch and discards it properly. Cleans the area with mild soap and warm water. Rinses area well and pats dry.		
17. Provides for the individual's safety. Returns the individual to a comfortable position.		
18. Cares for equipment and supplies.		
19. Removes gloves. Washes hands.		
20. Documents administration of the medication correctly. Compares the pharmacy label to the medication sheet a third time.		
21. Observes the individual for any unpleasant or harmful effects from the medication.		
22. Keeps medication storage areas locked at appropriate times and does not leave the areas unlocked when unattended.		

SKILL CHECKLIST

Procedure 7-7 Administration of Rectal Medications

Objective: To safely and effectively administer a rectal suppository, rectal gel, and rectal cream.

Instructions to the Learner: Following the licensed health care provider orders transcribed onto the medication sheet, correctly administer the rectal medications as stated by your instructor.

Directions to the Instructor: Write an S or U to indicate a satisfactory or unsatisfactory performance.

PROCEDURAL STEPS	S OR U	COMMENTS
1. Identifies the right individual.		
2. Washes hands.		
3. Gathers appropriate equipment.		
4. Works in a well-lighted, quiet, clean area.		
5. Compares the medication sheet with the licensed HCP orders.		
6. Identifies the right medication and removes the medication from the storage area.		
7. Checks the expiration date.		
8. Compares the pharmacy label to the medication sheet.		
9. Prepares the right dose (a and/or b):		
a. rectal suppository		
b. rectal cream and/or gel		
10. Compares the pharmacy label to the medication sheet for the second time.		
11. Double-checks the medication sheet to make sure the medication is being given to the right individual.		
12. Properly carries the medication and equipment to the individual.		
13. Has the individual urinate and/or move his bowels.		
14. Provides privacy.		
15. Assists the individual into a comfortable position.		
16. Puts on gloves.		
17. Administers the medication by the right route. Inserts the medication past the sphincter muscle (about 1 inch) into the rectum.		
18. Holds the buttocks together for 3 to 5 minutes. Has the individual hold the medication in his rectum for as long as possible or per licensed HCP orders.		
19. Assists individual to the bathroom, if needed.		
20. Provides for the individual's safety. Returns the individual to a comfortable position.		
21. Cares for equipment and supplies.		
22. Removes gloves. Washes hands.		
23. Documents administration of the medication correctly. Compares the pharmacy label to the medication sheet a third time.		
24. Observes the individual for any unpleasant or harmful effects from the medication.		
25. Keeps medication storage areas locked at appropriate times and does not leave the areas unlocked when unattended.		

SKILL CHECKLIST

Procedure 7-8 Administration of Vaginal Medications

Objective: To safely and effectively administer a vaginal suppository, vaginal cream, and ointment.

Instructions to the Learner: Following the licensed health care provider orders transcribed onto the medication sheet, correctly administer the vaginal medications as stated by your instructor.

Directions to the Instructor: Write an S or U to indicate a satisfactory or unsatisfactory performance.

PROCEDURAL STEPS	S OR U	COMMENTS
1. Identifies the right individual.		
2. Washes hands.		
3. Gathers appropriate equipment.		
4. Works in a well-lighted, quiet, clean area.		
5. Compares the medication sheet with the licensed HCP orders.		
6. Identifies the right medication and removes the medication from the storage area		
7. Checks the expiration date.		
8. Compares the pharmacy label to the medication sheet.		
9. Prepares the right dose (a and/or b): a. vaginal suppository b. vaginal cream and/or ointment		
10. Compares the pharmacy label to the medication sheet for the second time.		
11. Double-checks the medication sheet to make sure the medication is being given to the right individual.		
12. Properly carries the medication and equipment to the individual.		
13. Has the individual urinate and/or move her bowels.		
14. Provides privacy.		
15. Assists the individual into a comfortable position.		
16. Puts on gloves.		
17. Administers the medication by the right route.		
18. Encourages the individual to remain lying down for half an hour after inserting the medication.		
19. Explains to the individual that she is not to use tampons. Has her wear a sanitary pad if she wants to.		
20. Provides for the individual's safety. Returns the individual to a comfortable position.		
21. Cares for equipment and supplies.		
22. Removes gloves. Washes hands.		
23. Documents administration of the medication correctly. Compares the pharmacy label to the medication sheet a third time.		
24. Observes the individual for any unpleasant or harmful effects from the medication.		
25. Keeps medication storage areas locked at appropriate times and does not leave the areas unlocked when unattended.		

SKILL CHECKLIST

Procedure 7-9 Administration of Medications by Inhaler

Objective: To safely and effectively administer medication with an inhaler.

Instructions to the Learner: Following the licensed health care provider orders transcribed onto the medication sheet, correctly administer the medication by inhaler as stated by your instructor.

Directions to the Instructor: Write an S or U to indicate a satisfactory or unsatisfactory performance.

PROCEDURAL STEPS	S OR U	COMMENTS
1. Identifies the right individual.		
2. Washes hands.		
3. Gathers appropriate equipment.		
4. Works in a well-lighted, quiet, clean area.		
5. Compares the medication sheet with the licensed HCP orders.		
6. Identifies the right medication and removes the medication from the storage area.		
7. Checks the expiration date.		
8. Compares the pharmacy label to the medication sheet.		
9. Prepares the right dose.		
10. Compares the pharmacy label to the medication sheet for the second time.		
11. Double-checks the medication sheet to make sure the medication is being given to the right individual.		
12. Properly carries the medication and equipment to the individual.		
13. Assists the individual into a comfortable position.		
14. Has the individual remove his dentures.		
15. Has the individual drink water prior to administering the medication.		
16. Administers the medication by the right route. Has the individual hold her breath for a count of 10 before breathing out.		
17. Provides for the individual's safety. Returns the individual to a comfortable position.		
18. Has the individual brush her teeth and rinse well with an oral rinse. Assists the individual, if needed.		
19. Cares for equipment and supplies.		
20. Washes hands.		
21. Documents administration of the medication correctly. Compares the pharmacy label to the medication sheet a third time.		
22. Observes the individual for any unpleasant or harmful effects from the medication.		
23. Keeps medication storage areas locked at appropriate times and does not leave the areas unlocked when unattended.		

SKILL CHECKLIST

Procedure (Optional) Use of a Small-Volume Nebulizer

Objective: To safely and effectively use a small-volume nebulizer to administer normal saline or medication.

Instructions to the Learner: Following the licensed health care provider orders, correctly use a small-volume nebulizer to administer normal saline or medication as stated by the instructor.

Directions to the Instructor: Write an S or a U to indicate a satisfactory (S) or unsatisfactory (U) performance.

PROCEDURAL STEPS	S OR U	COMMENTS
1. Identifies the right individual.		
2. Verifies the licensed HCP orders.		
3. Washes hands.		
4. Gathers appropriate equipment.		
5. Explains the procedure to the individual.		
6. Provides privacy.		
7. Puts on protective equipment, if needed.		
8. Sets up equipment. Connects the equipment to oxygen or a gas source. Sets parameters on small-volume nebulizer.		
9. Fills nebulizer with sterile normal saline or medication.		
10. Assists the individual into the proper position.		
11. Observes the individual's respiratory rate and depth.		
12. Begins treatment. Observes the individual during the treatment.		
13. Ends treatment when the medication or saline has been administered. Continues to observe the individual's respiratory rate and depth.		
14. Disconnects the equipment from the oxygen or gas source.		
15. Properly disposes of soiled tissue. Cleans the emesis basin, if needed.		
16. Cleans and stores the mouthpiece. Rinses the nebulizer with sterile water or sterile saline and dries it well.		
17. Provides mouth care as needed.		
18. Removes protective equipment. Washes hands.		
19. Returns the individual to a comfortable position.		
20. Documents per workplace policy.		

SKILL CHECKLIST

Procedure 8-1 Use of a Pulse Oximeter

Objective: To safely and effectively perform a pulse oximetry reading to obtain an oxygen saturation level.

Instructions to the Learner: Following the licensed health care provider orders, correctly perform a pulse oximeter reading and obtain an oxygen saturation level as stated by the instructor.

Directions to the Instructor: Write an S or a U to indicate a satisfactory (S) or unsatisfactory (U) performance.

PROCEDURAL STEPS	S OR U	COMMENTS
1. Identifies the right individual.		
2. Verifies the licensed HCP orders.		
3. Washes hands.		
4. Gathers appropriate equipment.		
5. Explains the procedure to the individual.		
6. Provides privacy.		
7. If possible, raises the bed to a safe and comfortable working height.		
8. Assists the individual into a comfortable position.		
9. Locates the sensor site to be used.		
10. Cleanses the sensor site with an alcohol wipe or soap and water. If necessary, removes nail polish or artificial nails.		
11. Applies the sensor correctly in the designated location.		
12. Attaches the sensor to the pulse oximeter unit.		
13. Turns the pulse oximeter unit on. Listens for the beep. Adjusts the volume to the desired level.		
14. Adjusts the alarm limits according to the licensed HCP orders.		
15. Compares the individual's pulse rate on the unit to the individual's actual pulse rate.		
16. Covers the sensor with a towel or sheet.		
17. Notes the percentage of oxygen saturation. Notifies the licensed HCP of the initial reading.		
18. If the bed was elevated, lowers the bed.		
19. Washes hands.		
20. Documents per workplace policy.		
21. Continues to monitor the individual's respiratory rate, pulse rate, and general appearance.		

SKILL CHECKLIST

Procedure 8-2 Changing a Humidifier Bottle

Objective: To safely and properly change a humidifier bottle.

Instructions to the Learner: Following the licensed health care provider orders, correctly change a prefilled humidifier bottle and a refillable humidifier bottle as stated by the instructor.

Directions to the Instructor: Write an S or a U to indicate a satisfactory (S) or unsatisfactory (U) performance.

PROCEDURAL STEPS	S OR U	COMMENTS
1. Identifies the right individual.		
2. Verifies the licensed HCP orders.		
3. Washes hands.		
4. Gathers appropriate equipment.		
5. Explains the procedure to the individual.		
6. Provides privacy.		
7. Removes the humidifier bottle from its package. If using a refillable bottle, makes sure the bottle has been washed and sterilized.		
8. Fills the bottle with sterile distilled water.		
9. Connects the bottle to the flow meter on the oxygen administration equipment. Tightens the bottle securely.		
10. Connects the cannula or mask to the humidifier bottle. Places the cannula or mask on the individual.		
11. Turns on the oxygen. Sets the flow rate per the licensed HCP order.		
12. Checks the pressure relief valve.		
13. Writes the date and time the humidifier bottle was changed and the UAP's initials on a sticker. Places the sticker on the humidifier bottle.		
14. Washes hands.		
15. Documents per workplace policy.		
16. Continues to monitor the individual to ensure that the humidifier bottle continuously bubbles.		

SKILL CHECKLIST

Procedure 8-3 Use of an Incentive Spirometer

Objective: To assist an individual to safely and effectively use an incentive spirometer.

Instructions to the Learner: Following the licensed health care provider orders, assist an individual to correctly use an incentive spirometer as stated by the instructor.

Directions to the Instructor: Write an S or a U to indicate a satisfactory (S) or unsatisfactory (U) performance.

PROCEDURAL STEPS	S OR U	COMMENTS
1. Identifies the right individual.		
2. Verifies the licensed HCP orders.		
3. Washes hands.		
4. Gathers appropriate equipment.		
5. Explains the procedure to the individual.		
6. Provides privacy.		
7. Demonstrates deep breathing.		
8. Assists the individual into a sitting position.		
9. Sets the pointer on the incentive spirometer at the level or point ordered by the licensed HCP.		
10. Properly instructs and guides the individual through use of the incentive spirometer. Repeats the action per the licensed HCP order.		
11. Properly disposes of soiled tissue. Cleans the emesis basin, if needed.		
12. Cleans and stores the mouthpiece.		
13. Provides mouth care as needed.		
14. Washes hands.		
15. Returns the individual to a comfortable position.		
16. Documents per workplace policy.		

SKILL CHECKLIST

Procedure 9-1 Administration of a Cleansing Enema

Objective: To safely and effectively administer a cleansing enema.

Instructions to the Learner: Following the licensed health care provider orders, correctly administer the cleansing enema as stated by the instructor.

Directions to the Instructor: Write an S or a U to indicate a satisfactory (S) or unsatisfactory (U) performance.

PROCEDURAL STEPS	S OR U	COMMENTS
1. Identifies the right individual.		
2. Verifies the licensed HCP orders.		
3. Washes hands.		
4. Gathers appropriate equipment.		
5. Prepares the equipment in the utility room or individual's bathroom.		
6. Properly carries the equipment to the individual. Places the equipment on a towel on the chair at the foot or side of the individual's bed.		
7. Explains the procedure to the individual.		
8. Has the individual urinate and/or move her bowels.		
9. Provides privacy.		
10. If possible, raises the bed to a safe and comfortable working height.		
11. Assists the individual into the proper position.		
12. Puts on gloves.		
13. Places a disposable pad on the bed under the individual.		
14. Lubricates the tube, if needed.		
15. Administers the enema solution. Inserts the tubing 2 to 4 inches into the rectum.		
16. Holds the container 12 to 18 inches above the level of the opening of the rectum while the enema solution flows slowly into the rectum and bowel.		
17. Once the enema solution has been administered, clamps the tubing and slowly removes the tubing from the rectum.		
18. Cleans the buttocks with toilet tissue. Properly discards the toilet tissue.		
19. If the bed is elevated, lowers the bed.		
20. Removes gloves.		
21. Assists individual to the bathroom, commode, or bedpan if needed.		
22. Provides for the individual's privacy and safety. Returns the individual to a comfortable position.		
23. Puts on gloves.		
24. Cares for equipment and supplies.		
25. Observes the results of the enema.		
26. Removes gloves.		
27. Washes hands.		
28. Documents administration of the enema correctly.		
29. Observes the individual for any unpleasant or harmful effects from the enema.		

SKILL CHECKLIST

Procedure 9-2 Administration of a Ready-to-Use (Prepackaged) Enema

Objective: To safely and effectively administer a ready-to-use (prepackaged) enema.

Instructions to the Learner: Following the licensed health care provider orders, correctly administer the ready-to-use (prepackaged) enema as stated by the instructor.

Directions to the Instructor: Write an S or a U to indicate a satisfactory (S) or unsatisfactory (U) performance.

PROCEDURAL STEPS	S OR U	COMMENTS
1. Identifies the right individual.		
2. Verifies the licensed HCP orders.		
3. Washes hands.		
4. Gathers appropriate equipment.		
5. Prepares the equipment in the utility room or individual's bathroom.		
6. Properly carries the equipment to the individual. Places the equipment on a towel on the chair at the foot or side of the individual's bed.		
7. Explains the procedure to the individual.		
8. Has the individual urinate and/or move her bowels.		
9. Provides privacy.		
10. If possible, raises the bed to a safe and comfortable working height.		
11. Puts on gloves.		
12. Assists the individual into the proper position.		
13. Places a disposable pad on the bed under the individual.		
14. Removes the tip from the enema container. Gently squeezes the container to make sure the tip is not damaged.		
15. Lubricates the container, if needed.		
16. Administers the enema solution. Inserts the tip of the container 2 inches into the rectum.		
17. Gently squeezes and rolls the enema container from the bottom.		
18. Once the enema solution has been administered, slowly removes the tip of the container from the rectum.		
19. Wipes the buttocks with toilet tissue. Properly discards the toilet tissue.		
20. Removes gloves.		
21. If the bed is elevated, lowers the bed.		
22. Assists individual to the bathroom, commode, or bedpan if needed.		
23. Provides for the individual's privacy and safety. Returns the individual to a comfortable position.		
24. Puts on gloves.		
25. Cares for equipment and supplies.		
26. Observes the results of the enema.		
27. Removes gloves.		
28. Washes hands.		
29. Documents administration of the enema correctly.		
30. Observes the individual for any unpleasant or harmful effects from the enema.		

SKILL CHECKLIST

Procedure 10-1 Administration of a Continuous Tube Feeding

Objective: To properly and safely administer a continuous tube feeding by gastrostomy or jejunostomy tube.

Instructions to the Learner: Following the licensed health care provider orders, properly and safely administer a continuous tube feeding via gastrostomy or jejunostomy tube as stated by the instructor.

Directions to the Instructor: Write an S or a U to indicate a satisfactory (S) or unsatisfactory (U) performance.

PROCEDURAL STEPS	S OR U	COMMENTS
1. Identifies the right individual.		
2. Verifies the licensed HCP orders.		
3. Washes hands.		
4. Gathers appropriate equipment.		
5. Provides privacy.		
6. Explains the procedure to the individual.		
7. Assists the individual into the proper position.		
8. If possible, raises the working area to a safe and comfortable working height.		
9. Checks the G-tube or J-tube to make sure the tube is in the correct position.		
10. Properly prepares the formula. Correctly fills the formula bag and tubing.		
11. Puts on gloves.		
12. Checks for any signs or symptoms of infection or bleeding. If ordered by the licensed HCP, rotates the tube.		
13. Correctly flushes the G-tube or J-tube.		
14. Properly connects the tubing from the formula bag to the G-tube or J-tube.		
15. Correctly sets up the pump. Sets the flow rate per the licensed HCP order. Makes sure the alarm is set.		
16. Opens the clamp on the tubing. Turns on the pump. Presses start/run button.		
17. Removes gloves.		
18. If the work area was elevated, lowers the area.		
19. Monitors the feeding as needed.		
20. When the feeding has been administered, turns off the pump.		
21. Washes hands.		
22. Puts on gloves.		
23. Properly disconnects the tubing and formula bag.		
24. Correctly flushes the G-tube or J-tube. Reinserts the plug into the G-tube or J-tube.		
25. Leaves the individual in Fowler's position for at least 45 to 60 minutes.		
26. Cares for equipment and supplies.		
27. Removes gloves.		
28. Washes hands.		
29. Documents per workplace policy.		

SKILL CHECKLIST

Procedure 10-2 Administration of an Intermittent Feeding by Bolus

Objective: To properly and safely administer an intermittent tube feeding by bolus via gastrostomy or jejunostomy tube.

Instructions to the Learner: Following the licensed health care provider orders, properly and safely administer an intermittent tube feeding by bolus via gastrostomy or jejunostomy tube.

Directions to the Instructor: Write an S or a U to indicate a satisfactory (S) or unsatisfactory (U) performance.

PROCEDURAL STEPS	S OR U	COMMENTS
1. Identifies the right individual.		
2. Verifies the licensed HCP orders.		
3. Washes hands.		
4. Gathers appropriate equipment.		
5. Provides privacy.		
6. Explains the procedure to the individual.		
7. Assists the individual into the proper position.		
8. If possible, raises the working area to a safe and comfortable working height.		
9. Checks the G-tube or J-tube to make sure the tube is in the correct position.		
10. Properly prepares the formula. Correctly fills the formula bag and tubing.		
11. Puts on gloves.		
12. Checks for any signs or symptoms of infection or bleeding. If ordered by the licensed HCP, rotates the tube.		
13. Correctly flushes the G-tube or J-tube.		
14. Using a 60-mL (cc) syringe, correctly administers the amount of formula ordered by the licensed HCP.		
15. Correctly flushes the G-tube or J-tube. Reinserts the plug into the G-tube or J-tube.		
16. Leaves the individual in Fowler's position for at least 45 to 60 minutes.		
17. If the work area was elevated, lowers the area.		
18. Cares for equipment and supplies.		
19. Removes gloves.		
20. Washes hands.		
21. Documents per workplace policy.		

SKILL CHECKLIST

Procedure 10-3 Administration of an Intermittent Feeding by Gravity Drip Method

Objective: To properly and safely administer an intermittent tube feeding by gravity drip method via gastrostomy or jejunostomy tube.

Instructions to the Learner: Following the licensed health care provider orders, properly and safely administer an intermittent tube feeding by gravity drip method via gastrostomy or jejunostomy tube.

Directions to the Instructor: Write an S or a U to indicate a satisfactory (S) or unsatisfactory (U) performance.

PROCEDURAL STEPS	S OR U	COMMENTS
1. Identifies the right individual.		
2. Verifies the licensed HCP orders.		
3. Washes hands.		
4. Gathers appropriate equipment.		
5. Provides privacy.		
6. Explains the procedure to the individual.		
7. Assists the individual into the proper position.		
8. If possible, raises the working area to a safe and comfortable working height.		
9. Checks the G-tube or J-tube to make sure the tube is in the correct position.		
10. Properly prepares the formula. Correctly fills the formula bag and tubing.		
11. Puts on gloves.		
12. Checks for any signs or symptoms of infection or bleeding. If ordered by the licensed HCP, rotates the tube.		
13. Correctly flushes the G-tube or J-tube.		
14. Properly connects the tubing from the formula bag to the G-tube or J-tube.		
15. Correctly sets the flow rate per the licensed HCP order by adjusting the tightness of the clamp on the tubing of the formula bag.		
16. Removes gloves.		
17. If the work area was elevated, lowers the area.		
18. Monitors the feeding as needed.		
19. When the feeding has been administered, closes the clamp.		
20. Washes hands.		
21. Puts on gloves.		
22. Properly disconnects the tubing and formula bag.		
23. Correctly flushes the G-tube or J-tube. Reinserts the plug into the G-tube or J-tube.		
24. Leaves the individual in Fowler's position for at least 45 to 60 minutes.		
25. Cares for equipment and supplies.		
26. Removes gloves.		
27. Washes hands.		
28. Documents per workplace policy.		

SKILL CHECKLIST

Procedure 10-4 Care of Gastrostomy and Jejunostomy Tubes

Objective: To properly and safely care for a gastrostomy and jejunostomy tube.

Instructions to the Learner: Following the licensed health care provider orders, correctly clean and care for a gastrostomy and jejunostomy tube.

Directions to the Instructor: Write an S or a U to indicate a satisfactory (S) or unsatisfactory (U) performance.

PROCEDURAL STEPS	S OR U	COMMENTS
1. Identifies the right individual.		
2. Verifies the licensed HCP orders.		
3. Washes hands.		
4. Gathers appropriate equipment.		
5. Provides privacy.		
6. Explains the procedure to the individual.		
7. Assists the individual into the proper position.		
8. If possible, raises the working area to a safe and comfortable working height.		
9. Checks the feeding tube to make sure the tube is in the correct position.		
10. Puts on gloves.		
11. If an old dressing is present, removes the old dressing. Checks for drainage.		
12. Checks for any signs or symptoms of infection or bleeding. If ordered by the licensed HCP, rotates the tube.		
13. If the incision is not healed, removes nonsterile gloves and puts on sterile gloves. Follows sterile technique.		
14. Washes the area around the tube with warm water and soap. Rinses the area well.		
15. Using the cotton-tipped swab, thoroughly cleans any crust or drainage.		
16. If the individual needs to have the dressing replaced, appropriately redresses the tube site.		
17. If the feeding tube is 12 inches or longer, secures the tube.		
18. If the work area was elevated, lowers the area.		
19. Cares for equipment and supplies.		
20. Removes gloves.		
21. Washes hands.		
22. Documents per workplace policy.		

SKILL CHECKLIST

Procedure 10-5 Flushing Gastrostomy and Jejunostomy Tubes

Objective: To correctly and safely flush a gastrostomy or jejunostomy tube.

Instructions to the Learner: Following the licensed health care provider orders, correctly and safely flush a gastrostomy or jejunostomy tube.

Directions to the Instructor: Write an S or a U to indicate a satisfactory (S) or unsatisfactory (U) performance.

PROCEDURAL STEPS	S OR U	COMMENTS
1. Identifies the right individual.		
2. Verifies the licensed HCP orders.		
3. Washes hands.		
4. Gathers appropriate equipment.		
5. Provides privacy.		
6. Explains the procedure to the individual.		
7. If possible, raises the working area to a safe and comfortable working height.		
8. Assists the individual into the proper position.		
9. Checks the G-tube or J-tube to make sure the tube is in the correct position.		
10. Puts on gloves.		
11. Checks for any signs or symptoms of infection or bleeding. If ordered by the licensed HCP, rotates the tube.		
12. Pinches off the G-tube or J-tube.		
13. Removes the plug from G-tube or J-tube. Places the plug on a clean paper towel or in an emesis basin.		
14. Removes plunger from a 60-mL (cc) syringe. Inserts syringe (without plunger) into G-tube or J-tube.		
15. Fills syringe with warm water. Unpinches tube. Allows water to flow slowly from syringe through G-tube or J-tube into stomach or small bowel.		
16. Does not force water through G-tube or J-tube.		
17. Before syringe completely empties, pinches off G-tube or J-tube. Removes syringe from tube. Reinserts plug.		
18. Leaves the individual in Fowler's position for at least 45 to 60 minutes.		
19. If the work area was elevated, lowers the area.		
20. Cares for equipment and supplies.		
21. Removes gloves.		
22. Washes hands.		
23. Documents per workplace policy.		

SKILL CHECKLIST

Procedure 10-6 Checking for Residual Feeding

Objective: To accurately and safely check for residual feeding.

Instructions to the Learner: Following the licensed health care provider orders, accurately and safely check for residual feeding.

Directions to the Instructor: Write an S or a U to indicate a satisfactory (S) or unsatisfactory (U) performance.

PROCEDURAL STEPS	S OR U	COMMENTS
1. Identifies the right individual.		
2. Verifies the licensed HCP orders.		
3. Washes hands.		
4. Gathers appropriate equipment.		
5. Provides privacy.		
6. Explains the procedure to the individual.		
7. If possible, raises the working area to a safe and comfortable working height.		
8. Assists the individual into the proper position.		
9. Checks the G-tube or J-tube to make sure the tube is in the correct position.		
10. Puts on gloves.		
11. Checks for any signs or symptoms of infection or bleeding. If ordered by the licensed HCP, rotates the tube.		
12. Stops the feeding.		
13. Pinches off the G-tube or J-tube.		
14. Removes the tubing of the formula bag from the G-tube or J-tube. Caps the tubing. Places the tubing on a clean paper towel or hangs it over the pump.		
15. Inserts syringe with plunger into G-tube or J-tube.		
16. Gently pulls back the plunger of the syringe, allowing the contents of the stomach or small bowel to enter the syringe.		
17. If the amount of contents entering the syringe is less than 100 mL (cc), immediately pushes the contents back into the stomach or small bowel. Flushes the G-tube or J-tube. Restarts the feeding.		
18. If the total contents removed are greater than 100 mL (cc), returns all of the contents to the stomach or small bowel. Flushes the G-tube or J-Tube. Does not restart the feeding. Waits 30 to 60 minutes. Rechecks the residual.		
19. If the total contents are still greater than 100 mL (cc), again returns the contents to the stomach or small bowel. Flushes the G-tube or J-tube. Does not start the feeding. Immediately notifies the individual's licensed HCP and the supervisor.		
20. If the total contents are less than 100 mL (cc), returns the contents to the stomach or small bowel. Flushes the tube. Inserts the tubing of the formula bag. Restarts the feeding.		
21. Leaves the individual in Fowler's position.		
22. If the work area was elevated, lowers the area.		
23. Cares for equipment and supplies.		
24. Removes gloves.		
25. Washes hands.		
26. Documents per workplace policy.		

SKILL CHECKLIST

Procedure 10-7 Administration of Medication through a Gastrostomy or Jejunostomy Tube with a Continuous Feeding

Objective: To correctly and safely administer medication by gastrostomy or jejunostomy tube when an individual is receiving a continuous tube feeding.

Instructions to the Learner: Following the licensed health care provider orders, correctly and safely administer medication by bolus via gastrostomy or jejunostomy tube when an individual is receiving a continuous tube feeding.

Directions to the Instructor: Write an S or a U to indicate a satisfactory (S) or unsatisfactory (U) performance.

PROCEDURAL STEPS	S OR U	COMMENTS
1. Identifies the right individual.		
2. Verifies the licensed HCP orders.		
3. Washes hands.		
4. Gathers appropriate equipment.		
5. Prepares the medication per the licensed HCP orders.		
6. Provides privacy.		
7. Explains the procedure to the individual.		
8. If possible, raises the working area to a safe and comfortable working height.		
9. Assists the individual into the proper position.		
10. Checks the G-tube or J-tube to make sure the tube is in the correct position.		
11. Puts on gloves.		
12. Checks for any signs or symptoms of infection or bleeding. If ordered by the licensed HCP, rotates the tube.		
13. Stops the feeding. Shuts off the pump.		
14. Pinches the G-tube or J-tube. Removes the tubing of the formula bag from the G-tube or J-tube. Caps the tubing. Places the tubing on a clean paper towel or hangs the tubing over the pump.		
15. Inserts the plug into the G-tube or J-tube if needed and waits the required amount of time before administering medication.		
16. Flushes the G-tube or J-tube with 50 mL (cc) of warm water.		
17. Administers the correct amount of medication(s) ordered by the licensed HCP.		
18. Flushes the G-tube or J-tube with 50 mL (cc) of warm water.		
19. If needed, inserts the plug into the G-tube or J-tube and waits the required amount of time before restarting the feeding.		
20. Reconnects the tubing of the formula bag. Restarts the pump.		
21. Leaves the individual in Fowler's position.		
22. If the work area was elevated, lowers the area.		
23. Cares for equipment and supplies.		
24. Removes gloves.		
25. Washes hands.		
26. Documents per workplace policy.		

SKILL CHECKLIST

Procedure 10-8 Administration of Medication through a Gastrostomy or Jejunostomy Tube with an Intermittent Feeding

Objective: To correctly and safely administer medication by gastrostomy or jejunostomy tube when an individual is receiving an intermittent tube feeding.

Instructions to the Learner: Following the licensed health care provider orders, correctly and safely administer medication by bolus via gastrostomy or jejunostomy tube when an individual is receiving an intermittent tube feeding.

Directions to the Instructor: Write an S or a U to indicate a satisfactory (S) or unsatisfactory (U) performance.

PROCEDURAL STEPS	S OR U	COMMENTS
1. Identifies the right individual.		
2. Verifies the licensed HCP orders.		
3. Washes hands.		
4. Gathers appropriate equipment.		
5. Prepares the medication per the licensed HCP orders.		
6. Provides privacy.		
7. Explains the procedure to the individual.		
8. If possible, raises the working area to a safe and comfortable working height.		
9. Assists the individual into the proper position.		
10. Checks the G-tube or J-tube to make sure the tube is in the correct position.		
11. If the medications are ordered at the same times as the feedings, gives the medications at either the beginning or at the end of the feeding.		
12. If administering Dilantin, administers the medication at the appropriate interval to the feeding.		
13. Puts on gloves.		
14. Checks for any signs or symptoms of infection or bleeding. If ordered by the licensed HCP, rotates the tube.		
15. Pinches the G-tube or J-tube. Removes the plug from the tube. Places the plug on a clean paper towel or in the emesis basin.		
16. Removes the plunger from the syringe. Inserts the syringe without the plunger into the G-tube or J-tube. Unpinches the tube.		
17. Flushes the G-tube or J-tube with 50 mL (cc) of warm water.		
18. Administers the correct amount of medication(s) ordered by the licensed HCP.		
19. Flushes the G-tube or J-tube with 50 mL (cc) of warm water.		
20. Pinches the G-tube or J-tube. Removes the syringe. Reinserts the plug into the tube.		
21. Leaves the individual in Fowler's position for at least 45 to 60 minutes.		
22. If the work area was elevated, lowers the area.		
23. Cares for equipment and supplies.		
24. Removes gloves.		
25. Washes hands.		
26. Documents per workplace policy.		

SKILL CHECKLIST

Procedure 11-1 Administration of an EpiPen Auto-Injector

Objective: To safely and effectively administer an EpiPen Auto-Injector.

Instructions to the Learner: Following the licensed health care provider orders transcribed onto the medication sheet, correctly administer an EpiPen Auto-Injector as stated by the instructor.

Directions to the Instructor: Write an S or a U to indicate a satisfactory (S) or unsatisfactory (U) performance.

PROCEDURAL STEPS	S OR U	COMMENTS
1. When arriving at work and before an emergency arises:		
a. compares the medication sheet, pharmacy label, and licensed HCP order for use of the EpiPen		
b. checks the expiration date on the EpiPen		
c. checks the medication for discoloration		
2. When an emergency arises, identifies the right individual.		
3. Obtains the EpiPen.		
4. Grasps the EpiPen with the black tip pointing downward.		
5. Forms a fist around the EpiPen. Makes sure the black tip of the EpiPen is down.		
6. With the other hand, pulls off the gray activation cap from the EpiPen.		
7. Holds the black tip near the individual's thigh. Swings the EpiPen and jabs it firmly into the individual's outer thigh at a 90-degree angle to the thigh.		
8. Holds the EpiPen firmly in place for 10 seconds.		
9. Removes the EpiPen. Massages the area for several seconds.		
10. Checks the black tip. (If the needle is showing, the medication has been administered. If the needle is not showing, the medication has not been administered.) If the medication has not been administered, repeats steps 7 through 9.		
11. Bends the needle back against a hard surface. Puts the syringe-needle unit back into its carrying case. Recaps the carrying case. Discards the unit at the earliest possible time into a sharps container.		
12. Calls 911. Keeps the individual warm and avoids unnecessary movement. Immediately transports the individual to the nearest emergency medical care center.		
13. Informs the health care professionals that the individual has had an injection of epinephrine.		
14. If the EpiPen has not yet been discarded, gives it to the staff at the emergency medical care center to discard.		
15. Contacts the individual's licensed health care provider and the supervisor.		
16. Upon return to the workplace, documents per workplace policy.		

SKILL CHECKLIST

Procedure 33-1 Taking an Oral Temperature with an Electronic or Digital Thermometer

Objective: To accurately measure oral temperature using an electronic or digital thermometer.

Instructions to the Learner: Perform the task below as per the directions of your instructor.

Directions to the Instructor: Write an S or U to indicate a satisfactory or unsatisfactory performance.

PROCEDURAL STEPS	S OR U	COMMENTS
1. Gathers equipment.		
2. Washes hands.		
3. Identifies the individual.		
4. Provides privacy.		
5. Explains the procedure to the individual. Answers any questions.		
6. Asks the individual if she has had anything to eat or drink or has smoked within the last 15 minutes. If yes, waits 15 minutes before taking the temperature.		
7. If appropriate, puts on gloves.		
8. Covers the probe with a disposable cover.		
9. Inserts the probe appropriately.		
10. Holds the probe in position. Asks the individual to close her mouth and breathe through her nose.		
11. When the buzzer signals that the temperature has been reached, reads the temperature. Removes the probe.		
12. Throws the sheath cover in the trash. If wearing gloves, removes them and throws them in the trash.		
13. Returns the probe to its position in the thermometer case.		
14. Assists the individual in resuming prior activities.		
15. Washes hands.		
16. Writes the individual's temperature in the notes or on a notepad.		
17. Returns the thermometer to its charger.		

SKILL CHECKLIST

Procedure 33-2 Taking a Rectal Temperature with an Electronic or Digital Thermometer

Objective: To accurately measure rectal temperature using an electronic or digital thermometer.

Instructions to the Learner: Perform the task below as per the directions of your instructor.

Directions to the Instructor: Write an S or U to indicate a satisfactory or unsatisfactory performance.

PROCEDURAL STEPS	S OR U	COMMENTS
1. Gathers equipment.		
2. Washes hands.		
3. Identifies the individual.		
4. Provides privacy.		
5. Explains the procedure to the individual. Answers any questions.		
6. Lowers the back of the bed so that the individual is lying flat. Turns the individual onto her side.		
7. Puts on gloves.		
8. Covers the probe with a disposable cover. Applies a small amount of water-soluble lubricant to the tip of the sheath.		
9. Inserts the probe appropriately.		
10. Holds the probe in position.		
11. When the buzzer signals that the temperature has been reached, reads the temperature. Removes the probe.		
12. Throws the sheath cover in the trash. Removes gloves. Throws the gloves in the trash.		
13. Returns the probe to its position in the thermometer case.		
14. Assists the individual in resuming prior activities.		
15. Washes hands.		
16. Writes the individual's temperature in the notes or on a notepad.		
17. Returns the thermometer to its charger.		

SKILL CHECKLIST

Procedure 33-3 Taking an Axillary Temperature with an Electronic or Digital Thermometer

Objective: To accurately measure axillary temperature using an electronic or digital thermometer.

Instructions to the Learner: Perform the task below as per the directions of your instructor.

Directions to the Instructor: Write an S or U to indicate a satisfactory or unsatisfactory performance.

PROCEDURAL STEPS	S OR U	COMMENTS
1. Gathers equipment.		
2. Washes hands.		
3. Identifies the individual.		
4. Provides privacy.		
5. Explains the procedure to the individual. Answers any questions.		
6. If appropriate, puts on gloves.		
7. Wipes the axillary area clean.		
8. Covers the probe with a disposable cover.		
9. Places the probe appropriately. Keeps the individual's arm close to her body.		
10. Holds the probe in position.		
11. When the buzzer signals that the temperature has been reached, reads the temperature. Removes the probe.		
12. Throws the sheath cover in the trash. Removes gloves. Throws the gloves in the trash.		
13. Returns the probe to its position in the thermometer case.		
14. Assists the individual in resuming prior activities.		
15. Washes hands.		
16. Writes the individual's temperature in the notes or on a notepad.		
17. Returns the thermometer to its charger.		

SKILL CHECKLIST

Procedure 33-4 Taking a Temperature with a Tympanic Thermometer

Objective: To accurately measure temperature using a tympanic thermometer.

Instructions to the Learner: Perform the task below as per the directions of your instructor.

Directions to the Instructor: Write an S or U to indicate a satisfactory or unsatisfactory performance.

PROCEDURAL STEPS	S OR U	COMMENTS
1. Gathers equipment.		
2. Washes hands.		
3. Identifies the individual.		
4. Provides privacy.		
5. Explains the procedure to the individual. Answers any questions.		
6. Covers the probe with a disposable cover.		
7. Selects the correct setting on the thermometer.		
8. Puts on gloves, if appropriate.		
9. Positions the individual correctly.		
10. Gently pulls the top of the ear up and back.		
11. Places the probe correctly.		
12. Quickly presses the button to measure the temperature.		
13. When the buzzer signals that the temperature has been reached, removes the probe. Reads the temperature.		
14. Throws the sheath cover in the trash. Removes gloves. Throws the gloves in the trash.		
15. Assists the individual in resuming prior activities.		
16. Washes hands.		
17. Writes the individual's temperature in the notes or on a notepad.		
18. Returns the thermometer to its charger or turns the thermometer off.		

SKILL CHECKLIST

Procedure 33-5 Counting a Radial Pulse

Objective: To accurately obtain a radial pulse.

Instructions to the Learner: Perform the task below as per the directions of your instructor.

Directions to the Instructor: Write an S or U to indicate a satisfactory or unsatisfactory performance.

PROCEDURAL STEPS	S OR U	COMMENTS
1. Gathers equipment.		
2. Washes hands.		
3. Identifies the individual.		
4. Provides privacy.		
5. Explains the procedure to the individual. Answers any questions.		
6. Assists the individual into a comfortable position.		
7. Locates the radial pulse.		
8. Counts the beats for 60 seconds or 1 minute. Notes whether it is regular or irregular.		
9. Assists the individual in resuming prior activities.		
10. Washes hands.		
11. Writes the individual's radial pulse in the notes or on a notepad.		

SKILL CHECKLIST

Procedure (Optional) Counting an Apical Pulse

Objective: To accurately obtain an apical pulse.

Instructions to the Learner: Perform the task below as per the directions of your instructor.

Directions to the Instructor: Write an S or U to indicate a satisfactory or unsatisfactory performance.

PROCEDURAL STEPS	S OR U	COMMENTS
1. Gathers equipment.		
2. Washes hands.		
3. Identifies the individual.		
4. Provides privacy.		
5. Explains the procedure to the individual. Answers any questions.		
6. Assists the individual into a comfortable position.		
7. Wipes the earpieces and diaphragm of the stethoscope with alcohol before using the stethoscope.		
8. Counts the apical pulse for 60 seconds or 1 minute. Notes whether it is regular or irregular		
9. Assists the individual in resuming prior activities.		
10. Wipes the earpieces and diaphragm of the stethoscope with alcohol after using the stethoscope.		
11. Washes hands.		
12. Writes the individual's apical pulse in the notes or on a notepad.		

SKILL CHECKLIST

Procedure 33-6 Counting Respirations

Objective: To accurately count respirations.

Instructions to the Learner: Perform the task below as per the directions of your instructor.

Directions to the Instructor: Write an S or U to indicate a satisfactory or unsatisfactory performance.

PROCEDURAL STEPS	S OR U	COMMENTS
1. Gathers equipment.		
2. Washes hands.		
3. Identifies the individual.		
4. Provides privacy.		
5. Explains the procedure to the individual. Answers any questions.		
6. Assists the individual into a comfortable position.		
7. Locates the radial pulse.		
8. After counting the pulse, counts the number of respirations for 60 seconds or 1 minute. Notes the depth and regularity.		
9. Assists the individual in resuming prior activities.		
10. Washes hands.		
11. Writes the individual's respirations in the notes or on a notepad.		

SKILL CHECKLIST

Procedure 33-7 Measuring Blood Pressure with a Sphygmomanometer and Stethoscope

Objective: To accurately measure blood pressure using a sphygmomanometer and stethoscope.

Instructions to the Learner: Perform the task below as per the directions of your instructor.

Directions to the Instructor: Write an S or U to indicate a satisfactory or unsatisfactory performance.

PROCEDURAL STEPS	S OR U	COMMENTS
1. Gathers equipment.		
2. Washes hands.		
3. Identifies the individual.		
4. Provides privacy.		
5. Explains the procedure to the individual. Answers any questions.		
6. Assists the individual into a comfortable position.		
7. Has the individual rest for 3 minutes before taking her blood pressure.		
8. Wipes the earpieces and diaphragm of the stethoscope with alcohol before using the stethoscope.		
9. Selects the correct size blood pressure cuff and applies the cuff properly.		
10. Positions the individual's arm.		
11. Locates the brachial artery.		
12. Correctly measures the blood pressure.		
13. Writes the individual's blood pressure reading in the notes or on a notepad. Also writes down which arm was used and if the individual was lying, sitting, or standing.		
14. Assists the individual in resuming prior activities.		
15. Wipes the earpieces and diaphragm of the stethoscope with alcohol after using the stethoscope.		
16. Cares for equipment and supplies.		
17. Washes hands.		

SKILL CHECKLIST

Procedure 33-8 Measuring Blood Pressure with an Electronic or Automatic Blood Pressure Unit

Objective: To accurately measure blood pressure using an electronic or automatic blood pressure unit.

Instructions to the Learner: Perform the task below as per the directions of your instructor.

Directions to the Instructor: Write an S or U to indicate a satisfactory or unsatisfactory performance.

PROCEDURAL STEPS	S OR U	COMMENTS
1. Gathers equipment.		
2. Washes hands.		
3. Identifies the individual.		
4. Provides privacy.		
5. Explains the procedure to the individual. Answers any questions.		
6. Assists the individual into a comfortable position.		
7. Has the individual rest for 3 minutes before taking her blood pressure.		
8. Positions the individual's arm correctly.		
9. Locates the brachial artery.		
10. Selects the correct size blood pressure cuff and applies the cuff properly.		
11. If the machine has frequency control, sets control correctly.		
12. If the machine has an inflation control switch, sets switch correctly.		
13. Correctly measures the blood pressure.		
14. When the measurement is complete, reads the blood pressure.		
15. Writes the individual's blood pressure reading in the notes or on a notepad. Also writes down which arm was used and if the individual was lying, sitting, or standing.		
16. Assists the individual in resuming prior activities.		
17. Cares for equipment and supplies.		
18. Washes hands.		

SKILL CHECKLIST

Procedure 34-1 Administration of Diastat (Diazepam)

Objective: To safely and effectively administer Diastat gel (diazepam) rectally.

Instructions to the Learner: Following the licensed health care provider orders correctly transcribed onto the medication sheet, correctly administer Diastat gel (diazepam) rectally as stated by the instructor.

Directions to the Instructor: Write an S or a U to indicate a satisfactory (S) or unsatisfactory (U) performance.

PROCEDURAL STEPS	S OR U	COMMENTS
1. When arriving at work and before an emergency arises: a. compares the medication sheet, pharmacy label, and licensed HCP order b. checks the expiration date		
2. When an emergency arises, identifies the right individual.		
3. Assists the individual to a safe area away from objects. Protects his head.		
4. Obtains the Diastat, gloves, and water-soluble gel.		
5. Provides privacy.		
6. Removes the syringe from the box.		
7. Removes the protective cover from the syringe.		
8. Puts on gloves.		
9. Removes the individual's clothing.		
10. Lubricates the rectal tip of the syringe with water-soluble gel.		
11. Positions the individual properly.		
12. Separates the buttocks. Inserts the lubricated tip of the syringe gently into the rectum past the sphincter muscle, about 1 inch.		
13. Gently pushes the plunger of the syringe while slowly counts to 3. Stops once all of the medication has entered the rectum.		
14. Holds the syringe in place while slowly counts to 3, then removes the syringe from the rectum.		
15. Holds the buttocks together and counts slowly to 3.		
16. Redresses the individual.		
17. Leaves the individual in a comfortable position on his side. Provides for the individual's safety.		
18. Cares for equipment.		
19. Removes gloves.		
20. Washes hands.		
21. Documents per workplace policy.		
22. Observes the individual.		

NOTES